Nursing - Trends and Developments

Edited by Sandra Xavier and Lucília Nunes

Published in London, United Kingdom

Nursing - Trends and Developments
http://dx.doi.org/10.5772/intechopen.104162
Edited by Sandra Xavier and Lucília Nunes

Contributors
Almas Bandeali, Zeeba Maita, Beryl Juliet Sam, Zainab Attia Abdallah, Engy Abdel Rahman Khamis, Fatma M. Ibrahim, Ayiat Allah Wagdy Farag, Fernanda Loureiro, Vanessa Antunes, Zaida Charepe, Tiffany F. Kelley, Monika Ravik, Kristoffer Ravik Andresen, Wolter Paans, Mei-Yu Yeh, Hamidreza Haririan, Rosemeire Sartori de Albuquerque, Beatriz Aparecida Ozello Gutierreztwo, Christiane Borges do Nascimento Chofakian, Renata Figueiredo de Oliveira, Giovana Araújo de Moura, Eliane Ribeiro, Sandra Xavier, Lucília Nunes

First published in London, United Kingdom, 2024 by IntechOpen
IntechOpen is the global imprint of INTECHOPEN LIMITED, registered in England and Wales, registration number: 11086078, 5 Princes Gate Court, London, SW7 2QJ, United Kingdom

British Library Cataloguing-in-Publication Data
A catalogue record for this book is available from the British Library

Additional hard and PDF copies can be obtained from orders@intechopen.com

Nursing - Trends and Developments
Edited by Sandra Xavier and Lucília Nunes
p. cm.
Print ISBN 978-1-80356-428-9
Online ISBN 978-1-80356-429-6
eBook (PDF) ISBN 978-1-80356-430-2

For EU product safety concerns:
IN TECH d.o.o., Prolaz Marije Krucifikse Kozulić 3, 51000 Rijeka, Croatia,
info@intechopen.com or visit our website at intechopen.com.

Meet the editors

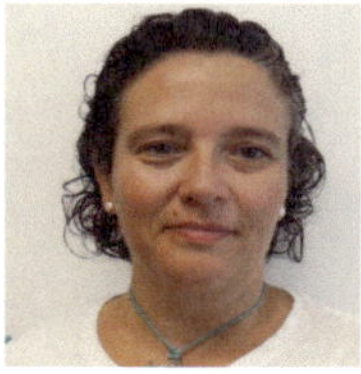

Sandra Xavier has diplomas in Community Mental Health and Nursing, a master's degree in Health Communication, a Ph.D. in Nursing, and a specialization in community nursing. She is a coordinator and professor in the Department of Community Health Nursing, Nursing School of Lisbon (ESEL), Portugal. She is also an integrated researcher at the Nursing Research, Innovation and Development Centre of Lisbon (CIDNUR).

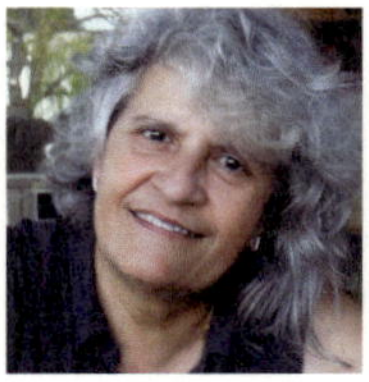

Lucília Nunes has aggregations in Nursing and Philosophy, master's degrees in Nursing Science and Cultural and Political History, and a Ph.D. in Philosophy. She is a professor in the School of Health, Polytechnic Institute of Setubal, Portugal, where she is also the coordinator of the Nursing Department. She is a member of the Ethics Committee of Setubal Hospital Centre and the Ethics Council of Minho University, Portugal. She is a founding member of the Portuguese Society of Nursing History.

Contents

Preface

We saw this book as a fertile soil for writing about research, practices, and concepts. The goal was to bring together different perspectives, preferably those that are "outside the box," innovative, and challenging, on what Nursing or perhaps tomorrow will look like.

The book's idea has been well-received by nurses, managers, researchers, and teachers around the world. There were more than 100 proposals and a wide range of themes, but the 11 chapters in this book stand out for their depth and quality, as well as their potential to be influential.

We depart from the conception that nursing is a discipline of knowledge and a profession that takes responsibility for continuous and evidence-based care of the sick and the dying as well as promoting the health of individuals, groups, families, and communities, helping them recover, rehabilitate, and reintegrate.

In addition to clinical practice, nurses are involved in patient advocacy, healthcare research, management, policy deliberation, higher education, and continuous training. Furthermore, nursing is the largest, most diverse, and most trusted profession in health care.

The State of The World's Nursing 2020 Report indicates that nursing is the largest occupation in the healthcare sector, comprising 59% of healthcare professionals. There are 27.9 million nurses in the workforce, of whom 19.3 million are professional nurses. Nearly half of healthcare workers are nurses and midwives, according to the WHO Director-General, who said the pandemic had reminded people "what incredible people are doing under incredible conditions." There are currently 27.9 million nurses in the world, which leaves 5.9 million short of what is needed.

In general, historians agree that Florence Nightingale was the catalyst for the development of professional and scientific nursing in the nineteenth century. As social, scientific, and technological changes, as well as the development and scientific legitimization of the profession have occurred since then, we have come a long way.

Nursing education has also evolved. Nurses are not recognized as much as they should be in many countries and contexts of care delivery. In spite of this, nurses have transformed hospitals, reorganized patterns of care to meet needs, brought care closer to homes and communities, and sought to mitigate inequalities.

As we reflect on the effects of the recent SARS-COV-2 pandemic (and likely in the future, as many consequences can be long-lasting, such as unredeemed bereavement), it becomes clear that nurses play a crucial role in crisis intervention, education, and literacy promotion.

There was also a change in the nursing education structure - nurses no longer had to rely on hospital-based training schools, higher education developed, and they were able to obtain a doctoral degree in nursing. A master's degree is typically required for specialized nursing practice or advanced nursing practice. In accordance with the International Council of Nurses (ICN), the scope of nursing practice "encompasses autonomous and collaborative care of individuals of all ages, families, groups, and communities, sick or well and in all settings."[1] By establishing practice standards and codes of ethics, national nursing associations clarify the scope of nursing practice.

The ICN has chosen the motto "*Our Nurses.Our Future*" for this year's International Nurse Day celebration. "Nurses provide care and leadership to address global health challenges everywhere, often at great personal risk. They are the essential life force for health, yet our healthcare systems worldwide have fallen short and failed to **value, protect, respect and invest** in this precious resource. The world has mistakenly taken nurses for granted, treating them as an invisible and inexhaustible resource. That must now stop for the sake of nurses and global health."[2]

The reflection on professional identity becomes evident when nurses ask themselves who they are, what they do, what specific characteristics the profession has, what goals they pursue, what activities they perform, what skills they develop, what is their purpose, what impact does it have on the care provided to people, how does it benefit their health? This territory is naturally plural, with forms of identity that differ, probably according to personal, social, and institutional identities, but come together in the shared statements about themselves and the dynamic nature of this social construction that converge. We are who we are because of the processes of professionalization and the paths of professionalism (understood as the development of competencies in the exercise of the profession throughout working life).

In addition to epistemology, ontology, ethics, hermeneutics, aesthetics, and deontology, nursing supports the professional identity, as well as science, technique, and praxis. We will all agree that nursing operates in health, in the healthcare spectrum, which both reports to population health, individual health and self-care, and primary and hospital healthcare – therefore is a liberal, self-regulated, higher educated profession. Every country in the world integrates the social mandate of the profession into the professional identity.

Our attention should be focused on the trends and developments occurring today in order to anticipate the future.

In order to fulfill this promise, we organized the 11 chapters into three sections, each serving as a potential challenge for nursing thought. We first introduce innovation and technology as approaches that can really raise debate and transform clinical

[1] International Council of Nurses. Definition of Nursing. In https://www.icn.ch/nursing-policy/nursing-definitions.

[2] International Council of Nurses. https://www.icn.ch/news/value-respect-protect-invest-icn-launches-international-nurses-day-posters.

practices in the section. A deeper understanding of teaching and learning processes can be gained in the second section. Furthermore, in the last section we have included other trends and developments, including general and diverse challenges related to management, clinical and health policy, and nursing.

Sandra Xavier, Ph.D.
Nursing School of Lisbon (ESEL),
Department of Community Health Nursing,
Nursing Research Unit for South and Islands [UIESI],
Lisbon, Portugal

CIDNUR - Nursing Research, Innovation and Development Centre of Lisbon,
Lisbon, Portugal

Lucília Nunes, Ph.D.
School of Health, Polytechnic Institute of Setúbal,
Nursing Department,
Setúbal, Portugal

NURSE'IN – UIESI Nursing Research Unit for South and Islands,
Setúbal, Portugal

Section 1

Inovation and Technology

Chapter 1

Advancing the Nursing Profession through Innovation

Tiffany F. Kelley

Abstract

To innovate is to bring forward positive change for a population of people who are affected by a pervasive unmet need. In nursing and healthcare, new innovations must address how to advance quality outcomes. These advancements can be through one or more of the six domains of quality *(e.g., safe, efficient, effective, equitable, timely, and patient-centered).* Nursing history is rich with innovation efforts to advance the profession. Nursing has recently experienced a new resurgence of focus on innovation through academics, practice, research, and scholarship. Nursing must continue to evolve and meet the contemporary needs of our peers and the people which we serve. Embracing the power of innovation as a profession can help us address the many pervasive unmet nursing and healthcare needs across the globe. This chapter will aim to: Define innovation, nursing, and healthcare innovation 1. Describe aspects of nursing innovation throughout history 2. Describe the role of quality as an outcome measure for innovation efforts 3. Examine how innovation can be a focal point in academics, practice, research, scholarship, and policy 4. Critique the risk of not embracing innovation in nursing and healthcare for the future.

Keywords: nursing, innovation, future of nursing, nursing advancements, innovations in healthcare

1. Introduction

The nursing profession has seen a growing focus on innovation over the last decade. Yet, more work remains to solidify innovation as a necessary learning element for the benefit of the care delivery and professional nursing contributions to individuals, families, groups, communities, and populations at large [1, 2]. Yet, innovation remains a new domain for many in nursing and healthcare. The purpose of this chapter is to describe how the nursing profession can advance through the integration of innovation into our knowledge, skills, and abilities across all areas where nurses work. The chapter is broken into five topical areas. Each topical area builds on the one(s) before it.

1.1 Chapter objectives

- Define innovation, nursing innovation and healthcare innovation.

- Describe aspects of nursing innovation throughout history.
- Describe the role of quality as an outcome measure for innovation efforts.
- Examine how innovation can be a focal point in academics practice research and scholarship.
- Critique the risk of not embracing innovation in nursing and healthcare for the future.

2. Define innovation, nursing innovation, and healthcare innovation

What does it mean to innovate, to be innovative, or to create an innovation? This is a common question for many when innovation is discussed in conversation. At times, innovation can lead to misconceptions, be seen as something ethereal (e.g., magic), be resisted, and may also be misunderstood. Innovation may be perceived by some as risky to healthcare while others may see it as the panacea for current challenges. In this section, innovation will be clearly defined and measurable for those reading along. By the end of the chapter, one will be confident in knowing that innovation can be taught. One can learn to innovate, be innovative, and develop an innovation for nursing and healthcare at large. The terms *innovation*, *nursing innovation*, and *healthcare innovation* are defined in this first section of the chapter.

Innovation is all around us in the marketplace, society, and how we interact with the world each day. Yet, it can be difficult to pinpoint innovation without a clear definition of the term. An *innovation* is often an outcome, but it can also be an action taken or process [3]. One can develop an innovation for use in the marketplace and society. One can also develop an innovative process for how something is done. Thus, the term can be used as a noun, adjective, and a verb. This chapter will primarily focus on innovation as an outcome.

Innovation *(defined)* is a new product, process, and/or service introduced into a marketplace or society that addresses an unmet need of a target population of people. This definition of innovation is purposely generic to apply to any industry. Innovations can be developed as new products, processes, and/or services.

A **product innovation** is often a tangible item. Something that takes a physical form. However, in the digital age, digital products are becoming more common. Product innovations may include *(but are not limited to)* the lightbulb, smartphone, or electric car. All three of these products were invented and innovated to address unmet needs of a population of people.

A **process innovation** is the way in which something happens or occurs. Process innovations may include *(but are not limited to)* step by step workflows and automated systems for how to do something. An example of a process innovation might be the adoption of mobile banking with digital photo deposits or video conferencing calls. While many are familiar with these process innovations today, they were not available in decades past. These process innovations changed the way in which people could complete their banking needs and/or complete their business needs.

A **service innovation** is something that is provided by a specialist to someone in need of that expertise. Service innovations may include *(but are not limited to)* the internet, email, and delivery services (e.g., food, goods, medications and more). The internet and email provided a new service for how to access information and communicate with others. Delivery services provided a new service to allow items to be sent to the recipient instead of the recipient having to pick up at the corresponding store. These service innovations created new options for people to complete activities of interest or need.

These new innovations emerge to address an *unmet need* that is experienced by a target population of people. An unmet need is a recognized gap that is experienced when trying to reach a desired goal or outcome. Below two examples of unmet needs are shared with examples of available innovative solutions today.

2.1 Example one: hard boiled egg

An example of an unmet need may be the desire to have a quick and easy way to peel a hard-boiled egg without making a mess and taking too much time. Peeling a hard-boiled egg often is frustrating to experience with little pieces of the shell breaking off as well as parts of the egg. An example of an innovative solution to this unmet need is the ability to purchase pre-peeled hard-boiled eggs (and avoid the egg peeling experience).

2.2 Example two: hanging a picture on the wall

Another example of an unmet need may be the desire to hang a picture on the wall. One needs a tool to be able to have the picture displayed on the wall. A hammer may serve as that tool to meet that need with a nail. While a hammer is not an innovation today, there was a time when it did not exist. A more recent innovation that addresses this unmet need would be double-sided tape that is designed for hanging pictures on a wall. This is a more recent innovation that avoids the need for a hammer and nail.

For an innovation to be successful, there must be a *target population of people* who are served by the innovation and are looking for the solution to their unmet need. The target population should be more than one person or a few people. The more people that are affected by the unmet need, the greater the impact of the innovation. Therefore, when considering an unmet need, clearly define who represents the target population of people and how many people are part of that target population.

2.3 Nursing and healthcare innovation

Now, the definition of innovation from above *(a new product, process and/or service introduced into a marketplace or society that addresses an unmet need of a target population of people)* can be applied to nursing and healthcare innovation. However, there are some additions to that definition. Nursing innovation makes innovation more specific to the discipline of nursing. The American Nurses Association [2] defines nursing as "the protection, promotion, and optimization of health and abilities; prevention of illness and injury; facilitation of healing; alleviation of suffering through the diagnosis and treatment of human response; and advocacy in the care of individuals, families, groups, communities, and populations". The science of nursing is grounded in caring for others and delivering high quality care. As a result, the definition of *nursing innovation* can be refined as a new product, process and/or service introduced into a marketplace or society that addresses an unmet need of a target population of people to support the delivery of quality nursing care.

Nursing innovations will also take on forms of new products, processes, and/or services. Some examples of nursing innovation products include the crash cart [4] and neonatal phototherapy [5]. A nursing innovation process example is the Wong-Baker Faces Pain Scale to evaluate pediatric pain [6]. Nursing innovation service examples include the American Red Cross [7] and the role of the Nurse Practitioner [8]. *(Section 3 describes several of these nursing innovations in more detail).*

Healthcare innovation has similarities to nursing innovation in definition. Healthcare is defined by the World Health Organization (WHO) as *"health is a state of complete physical, mental, and social well-being and not merely the absence of disease or infirmity"* [9]. With this guiding definition of healthcare and applying to innovation, *healthcare innovation* can be refined as a new product, process, and/or service introduced into a marketplace or society that addresses an unmet need of a target population of people to support optimal healthcare. Healthcare innovation incorporates nursing innovation into the scope and embraces the innovations of other healthcare disciplines *(e.g., medicine, pharmacy, allied health, and more)* and efforts.

Nursing and healthcare commonly rely on workarounds to address unmet needs that affect the ability to reach quality nursing and healthcare [10, 11]. Workarounds can take the form of products, processes, and/or services. Workarounds require innovative behaviors of others, but workarounds are not innovations. Workarounds are indicators of system, organizational, and/or societal unmet needs that need innovative solutions [10].

2.4 Theories of innovation

To further understand the concept of innovation, one must also be aware of the prominent innovation theories. The prominent innovation theories are grounded in business, economics, and sociology (to name a few). The prominent innovation theories help us understand how to look at innovation and become better at creating new innovations that can be explained by innovation theories. Eight prominent theories and the associated theorist are listed below. An original source for each of the theorists is provided as a reference for the reader.

- Jobs to be Done, Anthony Ulwick [12].
- Disruptive Innovation, Clayton Christensen [13].
- User Driven Innovation, Eric Von Hippel [14].
- Open Innovation, Henry Chesbrough [15].
- Free Innovation, Eric Von Hippel [16].
- Democratizing Innovation, Eric Von Hippel [17].
- Purposeful Innovation, Peter Drucker [18].
- Diffusion of Innovation, Everett Rogers [19].

3. Describe aspects of nursing innovation throughout history

Innovation looks into the future while history reflects on the past. These two may seem to be on opposite ends of the spectrum. However, they are interrelated disciplines. Reflecting on the past allows for us to influence the future. We can look back and see how innovations came to be, the problems they were solving, and the new problems that were introduced in need of newer solutions. Innovations are built on the past that is no longer meeting the needs of others.

For nursing, this is no different. Innovation is not new to nursing. From the very beginning of the profession and even leading up to it, nurses have innovated to meet the needs of others. However, the term innovation has not been as prominently used. Yet, the actions led to innovative developments to foster improved care, systems, tools and more for those who are in need. Those in need include patients, families, communities, and populations. One does not need to be a patient to need the care of nurses.

Innovations emerge through the minds, creativity, and resourcefulness of others. There was a time when nursing was not a profession. There was a time when we did not have resources that we depend on today to provide quality nursing care. Examples of such resources include nursing as a profession, public health nursing, the crash cart, nurse practitioners, simulation education tools, the American Red Cross, the stretcher, pediatric pain scale, neonatal phototherapy, and even the emergence of electronic health records has roots from a nurse. Each of the innovations mentioned above are briefly described below. The descriptions are organized according to either nursing roles or nursing resources for care.

3.1 Nursing professional roles

The science of caring is a foundation of the nursing profession [20]. The profession today consists of over 27 million nurses across the globe [21]. Yet, there was a time when a nurse emerged as a new professional role and educational career path. There are many nurses in history who have had a profound impact by innovating within the nursing profession. Florence Nightingale and Mary Seacole are two of those nurses. Florence Nightingale and Mary Seacole were both instrumental in supporting soldiers during the Crimean War [22]. Florence Nightingale's innovative efforts focused on is often referred to as the founder of modern-day nursing [23]. Nightingale had many contributions during the Crimean War however her efforts to connect sanitation, nutrition, and overall cleanliness on the health status of wounded soldiers were new contributions to nursing [24]. Mary Seacole also provided significant contributions during the Crimean War. Seacole, who was known by many as "Mother Seacole" identified many ways to support and positively impact the British troops. Seacole used her Jamaican herbal remedies to provide nursing care to the ill and wounded. Additionally, she created the British Hotel that served as a storehouse where British soldiers were able to get necessary food, medicine, and supplies. The contributions of Nightingale and Seacole during the Crimean War led to their acknowledgements as Crimean Heroines [25]. Innovation was inherent in their abilities as nurses. Throughout the profession's history, nurses have continued to exhibit innovativeness in their nursing contributions. The examples shared in this section are just a few of the many nurses who have created necessary innovations that are staples today.

3.1.1 Public health nursing

In March 2020, the whole world became very aware of the need for public health nurses and public health expertise. Public health nursing is defined by the American Public Health Association [26] as "the practice of promoting and protecting the health of populations using knowledge from nursing, social and public health sciences". With 8 billion people in the world [27] and the World Health Organization defining health as "the state of complete physical, mental, and social well-being and not merely the absence of disease or infirmity" [9] there absolutely is a need for public health nurses. The origins of public health nursing date back to 1893 and the innovativeness of Lillian Wald [28]. Lillian Wald was a nurse who advanced the nursing profession to establish the term public health nurse. Today, there are nearly 16,000 public health nurses in the United States.

3.1.2 Nurse practitioners

In 1965, the United States established Medicare and Medicaid. Medicare and Medicaid provided greater access to healthcare services for more people. With more access to care, there was a need for many more primary care providers. Loretta Ford, a nurse, and Henry Silver, a physician, got together and innovated to create a new provider role: the Nurse Practitioner [29]. At the time, there was a shortage of available pediatric primary care providers. The new provider role and educational experience led to the Pediatric Nurse Practitioner role. From that first Nurse Practitioner role, others began to emerge (e.g., Adult Primary Care, Family) for nurses to pursue. Today there are over 355,000 Nurse Practitioners in the United States [30].

3.2 Nursing innovations for care

As nurses are in a profession of caring. The actions of their efforts are directed toward others (either directly or indirectly). Those who are recipients of care experience the greatest health outcomes when care is of high quality (more on that in Section 4). To provide high quality care, nurses need appropriate resources and tools to address care needs. Anything that does not exist naturally in nature was created by an individual or a group of individuals. The impetus for creating new innovations, as mentioned in Section 2, stems from an unmet need affecting a target group of people. As nurses are the healthcare professional group who spend the most time with patients, they are also able to recognize gaps, or unmet needs, in available resources (or solutions) that could enhance their caregiving. A nurse is attributed to many nursing resources depended upon today that are staples of caregiving for nurses and the healthcare team at large. Those resources include, but are not limited to, the American Red Cross, simulation mannequins for education, the crash cart, the stretcher, electronic health records, and one of the most prominently used pediatric pain scale tools. Each mentioned innovation is briefly described below.

3.2.1 American red Cross

The American Red Cross was founded in 1881 in the United States. Clara Barton advocated for the United States to establish a Red Cross for some time before its inception. She led the organization for 23 years. Barton provided nursing care during the Civil War and earned herself the nickname of Angel of the Battlefield. In 1869, Barton went to Switzerland and learned of the Red Cross while there. She saw that America could benefit from an organization that provided resources to those injured and brought the idea to the U.S. Twelve years later, the American Red Cross was established in the U.S. Barton saw that America did not have a comparable resource to support people who were hurt or in need of aid because of the war. The American Red Cross recognizes Barton's innovative efforts that has sustains over 140 years, "because of one woman, Clara Barton, the American Red Cross brings help and hope across the nation and around the world." [31].

3.2.2 Simulation mannequin for nursing education

Nursing education today has advanced to include the use of simulation mannequins that can present clinical scenarios to students that they may not see while in their clinical rotations. The evolution of simulation in nursing education can be traced back to nurse A. Lauder Sutherland in 1910. Sutherland invented the first simulation mannequin that became known as Mrs. Chase at Hartford Hospital in Connecticut [32, 33]. Mrs. Chase is now on display at Hartford Hospital's Innovation Center. Today, simulation is a core learning experience of nursing education.

3.2.3 Crash cart

The modern-day crash cart was invented by Anita Dorr. In 1967, Anita Dorr was working in an Emergency Department. Dorr recognized the lack of efficiency and organization to gathering necessary supplies when patient emergency situations would occur. Dorr decided to work with her husband to develop the first crisis cart that was made out of wood. She painted it red and added wheels to the bottom for ease of transport to and from areas within the emergency department. The crisis cart supported more effective patient care. Her innovativeness and invention led to the staple nurses and healthcare professionals depend upon today, the modern-day crash cart. Every care area has a crash cart in the event of a patient emergency [4].

3.2.4 Stretcher

Stretchers are a common form of transporting a patient within a hospital or healthcare facility. The origins of the stretcher date back to 1926. The inventor and innovator, Elizabeth Kenney, was caring for patients during World War I. Kenney saw the need for a more comfortable and easy way to transport patients to minimize their suffering in transport. Today, stretchers are a necessary piece of equipment within hospitals and healthcare facilities [32, 34].

3.2.5 Wong-baker faces pain scale

Prior to 1983, there was not a systematic way for pediatric patients' pain to be communicated and measured to the nurse. Donna Wong, a registered nurse, and Connie Baker, a child life specialist, both saw the need for a better way to help these children and their pain. Through their collective innovative research, the Wong-Baker Faces Pain Scale was developed and put into practice. Today, the Wong-Baker Faces Pain Scale is used around the world with people over the age of 3 [35].

3.2.6 Electronic health records

Electronic health records (EHRs) date back to the 1950's. Harriet Werley was one of the first (if not the first) nurse to examine the possibility of using computer technology to support the use and management of healthcare data and information [35]. Despite the conceptualization and initial versions that emerged in the 1960's, EHRs did not reach near full adoption until the last few years [36, 37]. While EHRs continue to have areas for enhancement and refinement, digitizing healthcare data creates new opportunities for improving quality care [38].

The nursing profession has a rich history of nurses who exhibit innovative behaviors to create necessary innovations. The innovations shared in this section are just a few of the many innovations that nurses have created to contribute to the unmet needs of groups, communities, and populations for higher care quality.

4. Describe the role of quality as an outcome measure for innovation efforts

Reflecting on the definition provided at the start of the chapter, innovation is a new product, process, and/or service that addresses a pervasive unmet need for a population of people to support optimal healthcare quality. Innovations introduced into healthcare settings must work to improve care quality. Improving care quality is not necessarily a requirement for non-nursing and/or non-healthcare innovations. However, with regulatory requirements, ethical considerations, and more, nurse innovators will increase their likelihood of innovation adoption and use with clarity around how quality of care can be improved through the innovation.

4.1 Quality

In 2000, the Institute of Medicine (IOM) (now the National Academy of Medicine (NAM)) published the seminal report, Crossing the Quality Chasm [39]. Within that report, healthcare quality was defined as "the degree to which healthcare services for individuals and populations increase the likelihood of desired health outcomes and are consistent with current professional knowledge" [40]. More specifically, quality was broken into six different domains. The six quality domains are: safe, efficient, effective, equitable, patient-centered, and timely. Each attribute is defined below as described by the IOM (now NAM).

4.1.1 Safe

Safe care is care that is free from any unintended injury, harm, or error [40]. Nurses and healthcare professionals have an ethical expectation to provide care void of any intentional harm or negligence. While an ethical expectation, there are times when errors do occur. Therefore, one domain of quality is to promote and establish safe care practices, policies, and solutions to reduce the risk of unintended injury, harm, or error to others.

4.1.2 Efficient

Efficient care is care that avoids unnecessary waste and/or costs [40]. Unnecessary waste and/or costs could apply to tangible and intangible items. Tangible waste and/or costs could be medical supplies, exams, tests, procedures, and visits. Intangible waste could be unnecessary wait times, delays, and/or interruptions to care delivery. While not intentional, any lack of efficiency around the unnecessary waste and/or costs has room for improvement toward optimal care quality.

4.1.3 Effective

Effective care integrates evidence-based practice into the care delivery process [40]. Care delivery is largely evidence-based. The evidence-based protocols are based on research outcomes and analysis to determine the most effective procedures and protocols to achieve optimal health outcomes for the affected people. Yet, new evidence-based practice protocols and procedures evolve as patients' responses indicate the need for new tools to reach a desired outcome.

4.1.4 Equitable

Equitable care is care that is optimally delivered to all people, regardless of gender, ethnicity, geography, socioeconomic status, and more [40]. Every person is deserving of nursing and healthcare that is equitable. However, evaluation of one's social determinants of health may indicate that there are additional care needs to include and/or adjust to deliver equitable care.

4.1.5 Patient-centered

Patient-centered care focuses on individualizing care to the specific patient [40]. Every patient is a person who has personal preferences and clinical preferences for care [41]. Patients are people first with clinical and personal care needs. Patients want to be treated like a person and not a protocol or diagnosis. Patients have unique insights that must be considered for patient-centered care by nurses and healthcare professionals.

4.1.6 Timeliness

Timeliness of care is care that is delivered without delays [40]. Nurses and healthcare professionals aim to deliver care in a timely manner (void of delays). However, most nurses, healthcare professionals, and patients are aware of instances of delayed care. Delayed care could be the wait time for an available appointment, emergency room wait time and/or time to be admitted or discharged.

4.2 Quality influencing nursing and healthcare innovation

With these six domains of quality, innovators can begin to work backwards with the six domains of quality as the starting place for consideration and exploration of unmet needs affecting a population of users. The population of users could be nurses, patients, family members, groups, communities, all people and/or any other subgroup. The unmet need(s) to identify as an innovator is(are) gaps or limitations in care delivery related to at least one of the six domains: safe, efficient, effective, equitable, patient-centered, and timeliness.

To identify potential opportunities for innovation, consider where there are specific current gaps and/or limitations in care delivery. Once that gap and/or limitation is identified, consider what the implications are for care quality. Go back to the definitions above and identify how that gap and/or limitation is not fully fulfilling the expectation of the domain (or domains if more than one identified). By identifying the gap in quality through one or more of the domains, there is the opportunity to measure the impact of the gap and subsequently the impact of the forthcoming innovation. Next, use the principles of innovation theory and design thinking methodology [42] to formulate an idea and process to develop an innovative solution, prototype, and plan for bringing to the market and/or society.

5. Examples of gaps and/or limitations with possible innovative solution ideas

5.1 Safe

To experience safe care, people would experience care that is free from any unintended injury, harm, or error. Falls are a common unintended injury people experience. Over three million aging adults fall each year. Over eight hundred thousand are hospitalized because of a fall [43]. Preventing falls for safety becomes an unmet need. Therefore, one may begin to study the primary reasons why falls occur and determine an innovation to prevent falls that is not currently available.

5.2 Efficient

To experience efficient care, patients would experience care that removes or reduces unnecessary waste and/or costs. Frequently, patients may experience repetitive tests that are done at different healthcare facilities. However, that repetitive test will lead to increased overall healthcare costs. At times, the repeat test may be necessary. However, unnecessary repetitive tests lead to unnecessary healthcare costs [44]. Thus, one may be interested in investigating how to reduce the use of unnecessary repetitive tests for appropriate specificity and sensitivity.

5.3 Effective

Effective care integrates evidence-based practice into the care delivery process [40]. Care delivery is largely evidence-based. The evidence-based protocols are based on research outcomes and analysis to determine the most effective procedures and protocols to achieve optimal health outcomes for the affected people. Yet, new evidence-based practice protocols and procedures evolve as patients' responses indicate the need for new tools to reach a desired outcome. Evidence based innovation efforts have a cyclical relationship with evidence-based practice [45]. Yet, new knowledge from research does not tend to be translated to practice for approximately 17 years [46]. One may be interested in determining how to create a model for more seamless integration of new evidence-based innovation toward evidence-based practice in a more effective timeframe.

5.4 Equitable

Equitable care includes addressing social determinants of health. Social determinants of health include the categories of economic stability, education access and quality, healthcare access and quality, neighborhood and build environment, and social and community context. There are variables within each category to be measured. Social determinants of health are part of Healthy People 2030 [47]. One may be interested in exploring how best to either collect such data in an equitable way from people and/or determine how to use such data for creating new healthcare innovations that can contribute to enhanced equity across all care settings.

5.5 Patient-centered

Nurses and healthcare professionals cannot describe what patient-centered care means to patients unless one has also been a patient. To deliver patient-centered care, nurses and healthcare professionals must focus on providing individualized care. At times, patients may feel as though they are treated as a diagnosis or protocol rather than an individual person. This may not be the intention of the nurse or healthcare professional. Therefore, one may be interested in exploring how to reframe patient-centered care in such a way that patients feel known as people.

5.6 Timeliness

Delivering care in a timely manner, void of delays, is important to all. However, delays do occur. Delays in the time desired to obtain an appointment with a provider from the time requested, delays in the time seen when in an emergency department waiting room, and delays in time to discharge from a hospital or facility are three commonly experienced care delays. An innovator may seek to find ways to reduce such delays for the patient.

The examples are meant to offer a way to consider where to start on identifying possible areas for innovation. There are ample opportunities for innovation within healthcare. The more nurses, healthcare professionals, and people in general who opt to engage in innovation, the more advancements, improvements, and transformations nursing and healthcare will see in the future.

6. Examine how innovation can be a focal point in academics practice research, scholarship, and policy

Nursing and healthcare have persistent challenges that are in dire need of innovative solutions. Momentum for integrating innovation into the nursing profession as an active effort has continued to grow over the last decade across the globe. Through innovation, nursing, *(as a profession),* and healthcare, (*as an industry*), can further develop and advance for the benefit of individuals, families, groups, communities, and populations at large affected by the persistent and emerging unmet needs affecting quality nursing and healthcare. Innovation occurs through people. People must be knowledgeable on the principles of innovation and how to apply it to increase the likelihood of successful adoption within the marketplace and society.

People cannot be expected to successfully develop new nursing and healthcare innovations without knowing how to do so. Therefore, nurses can and must be taught about innovation as a concept, prominent theories, methodologies, and how to apply into practice and research. There are five domains where innovation can be a focal point for inclusion. The five domains are: academics, practice, research, scholarship, and policy.

6.1 Academics

To become a nurse, one must experience academic preparation. The nursing profession prepares registered nurses through undergraduate and graduate level education. Students can and must be academically prepared early in their academic nursing education on the foundational concepts, theories, and principles of innovation. Providing students with innovation education during undergraduate education will prepare future nurses with the tools to know how to create positive change as an innovation when faced with gaps in care (e.g., unmet needs). For those nursing students who opt to pursue graduate education, the foundational principles continue to be of importance as well as innovative leadership education (e.g., MS, DNP) and innovative research approaches that may lead to new discoveries (e.g., PhD). Additionally, there must be acknowledgement of the need for faculty preparation around nursing and healthcare innovation. Investing in the preparation of more faculty interested in or having an experiential background in innovation will provide a more effective experience for desired student outcomes.

6.2 Practice

Nursing roles are largely practice based across the globe. The public depends on nurses and healthcare professionals' commitment to their practice. Yet, there are often areas where there is room for innovation in the day-to-day nursing practice. Workarounds are unfortunately a common nursing practice that are often indicative of a larger organizational level gap. While workarounds require innovative behaviors, the impact of the workaround is for the "n" of 1. If necessary, one might need to redo the workaround again the next day or for the next patient. Innovations also require innovative behaviors however they solve for the "n" of many at scale. As a profession, nursing must recognize workarounds for their clues as to possible innovations needed for development [48]. Nursing must also recognize the need for nurses to shift their mindsets away from workarounds toward innovations. This will require the academic preparation as stated above but also a supportive culture of innovation within the practice settings where new ideas can be shared and considered for development. Innovation centers are an emerging supportive structure at hospitals and academic centers in the United States.

6.3 Research

Research is the discovery of new knowledge. Nursing science advances through conducting research studies to answer questions that remain unanswered about a particular phenomenon. The nursing profession and healthcare industry benefit from nursing research. While this chapter has largely focused on innovation as the outcome, innovative approaches to research may lead to novel outcomes. An innovative research approach may be reflected in the formed research question. Another innovative approach may be reflected in the methodological approach to the larger nursing issue. The approach could be in the methods used and/or the analysis of the data. With new or novel questions and/or approaches, the researcher may uncover new findings that contribute to the larger phenomenon. New findings may also reveal insights needed to determine a suitable innovation.

6.4 Scholarship

Scholarship is the way in which new knowledge is generated and disseminated for the greater good of society. Scholarship may include discovery, teaching, integration, and/or application [49]. Discovery is the action of generating new knowledge and insights for the profession. Teaching is the action of educating students on the knowledge, skills, and abilities necessary for course content area. Professors aim to scale their knowledge to others through the teaching process. The integration and application of the new knowledge and teachings into practice can be done in many forms as nurses and healthcare professionals.

Innovation is an emerging specialty discipline for the nursing profession. As innovation continues to grow in focus and scope, innovators can recognize that there are four areas of scholarship where more innovation efforts are needed for nursing. The profession needs more innovative discoveries to address the current and future challenges. Professors of innovation are needed to teach students the fundamentals of innovation concepts, theories, methodologies, and applications for effectiveness. Additionally, such students will be needed to scale the knowledge to others across the profession in the same way that the nurse practitioner role and education grew over time. Integration and application will mean that innovators and innovative cultures will emerge for changes to occur throughout the profession.

6.5 Policy

Health care is a highly regulated industry. Regulations determine what is legally permissible for healthcare delivery. Innovations can be advanced because of regulations or deterred to a potential future date. Additionally, healthcare costs are largely paid for by a third party (e.g., not the patient). In the United States, the Centers for Medicare and Medicaid Services (CMS), is the largest payer of healthcare services [50]. Payer reimbursements can also be influence positively or negatively depending upon whether a reimbursable service. In the United States, telehealth services became a reimbursable service in March 2020 with the onset of the coronavirus global pandemic [51]. Despite the conceptualization of telehealth in the 1960's [52], adoption had been slow prior to the pandemic due to challenges in a viable business model. Innovators must be aware of the state of regulatory opportunities and challenges when pursuing an innovation. Additionally, innovators must also become participants in the policy process to support the advancement of nursing and healthcare through their eyes on the future.

7. Critique the risk of not embracing innovation in nursing and healthcare for the future

As shared earlier in this chapter, innovation is not new to the nursing profession. Nurses have helped transform and advance the profession. Through their own innovative behaviors and innovation developments, nurses throughout history have identified unmet needs affecting others and the associated optimal health status. Their discoveries and advancements have helped propel nursing and healthcare forward. What was new at that time is now a staple of care delivery for the 21st century.

A difference between the past and the current moment for nursing is the active interest in innovation at a strategic professional level. While the word "innovation" may not always be present, the act of seeking to promote the creation of positive change for optimal health outcomes is indicative of the desire to innovate. Organizations such as the World Health Organization, the American Nurses Association, and the American Association of Colleges of Nursing (to name just a few) have all set forth efforts to foster the advancement of nursing [53–55]. As the health needs of people change and evolve, so will the products, processes, and services that are needed to provide optimal care quality.

Yet, nursing and healthcare has traditionally been slow to adopt change. A commonly used phrase is, "*we have always done it this way*". When that phrase is heard, the readers should consider that the process in question may not have been evaluated in some time. This may be an indication for a necessary exploration of potential change, improvement, and/or innovation. The reader can identify that phrase as an opportunity to explore the job to be done and how it may be able to be innovated for higher quality care.

One cannot expect transformational and impactful change to occur, without embracing innovation in nursing and healthcare for the future. To do so requires acknowledgement of the science of innovation and how nurses and healthcare professionals must have the innovation knowledge, skills, and abilities to be able to provide ideas, innovations, and a supportive culture to meet the unmet needs of the present and the future.

8. Conclusion

Ideally, nursing innovation will emerge as a formalized specialty practice within the nursing profession in the coming years. With a formalized specialty practice, the foundations can be established to create scalable pathways for nurses across the globe to make impactful contributions to nursing, healthcare, and society at large. Innovations occur through people. The more people who have the knowledge, skills, and abilities to innovate, the greater the likelihood for positive change within the nursing profession and healthcare industry. Until that does occur, the reader can feel confident in having the following knowledge from this chapter:

1. The ability to define innovation, nursing innovation, and healthcare innovation.

2. Describe several innovations created and invented by nurses throughout the profession's history.

3. Describe the role of healthcare quality for identifying unmet needs in innovation efforts.

4. Examine how innovation can be a focal point in academics, practice, research, scholarship, and policy.

5. Examine the risk of not embracing innovation in nursing and healthcare for the future.

DOI: http://dx.doi.org/10.5772/intechopen.110704

Acknowledgements

The author would like to acknowledge the University of Connecticut School of Nursing in their ongoing support and contributions to advance the nursing profession through innovation. The author would also like to acknowledge the innovation ecosystem within the University of Connecticut that has embraced the School of Nursing's ongoing innovation efforts. Lastly, the author would like to acknowledge the Frederick A. DeLuca Foundation for the support of this important work.

Conflict of interest

The author declares no conflict of interest.

Notes/thanks/other declarations

Thank you for the opportunity to contribute to this book.

Author details

Tiffany F. Kelley
University of Connecticut School of Nursing, Storrs, CT, USA

*Address all correspondence to: tiffany.kelley@uconn.edu

References

[1] Cusson R, Meehan C, Bourgault A, Kelley T. Educating the next generation of nurses to be innovators and change agents. Journal of Professional Nursing. 2020;**36**:13-19. DOI: 10.1016/j.profnurs.2019.07.004

[2] American Nurses Association. Scope of Practice. [Internet]. n.d. Available from: https://www.nursingworld.org/practice-policy/scope-of-practice/#:~:text=What%3A%20Nursing%20is%20the%20 protection,groups%2C%20communities%2C%20and%20populations. [Accessed: January 8, 2023]

[3] Barlow J. Managing Innovation in Healthcare. New Jersey: World Scientific; 2017

[4] Nelson R. Nursing innovation: Empowering nurses to solve workplace challenges using design thinking. American Journal of Nursing. 2020;**120**:18-19

[5] Bedi J. Sharon Ragone. [Internet]. 2021. Available from: https://invention.si.edu/node/28532/p/599-sharon-rogone. [Accessed: January 8, 2023]

[6] Wong-Baker Faces. Wong-Baker FACES History [Internet]. 2006. Available from: https://wongbakerfaces.org/us/wong-baker-faces-history/. [Accessed: January 7, 2023]

[7] Michals D. Clara Barton. [Internet]. 2015. Available from: https://www.womenshistory.org/education-resources/biographies/clara-barton. [Accessed: January 7, 2023]

[8] Berg JA. The perils of not knowing the history of the nurse practitioner role. Journal of the American Association of Nurse Practitioners. 2020;**32**:602-609

[9] World Health Organization. Constitution. [Internet]. 2022. Available from: https://www.who.int/about/governance/constitution. [Accessed: January 3, 2023]

[10] Kelley T, Brandon D, McGrath J. Workarounds as a catalyst to drive a culture of innovation in neonatal care. Advances in Neonatal Care. 2018;**18**:163-164. DOI: 10.1097/anc.0000000000000517

[11] Tucker AL, Heisler WS, Janisse LD. Designed for workarounds: A qualitative study for the causes of operational failures in hospitals. The Permanete Journal. 2014;**18**:33-41. DOI: 10.7812/TPP/13-141

[12] Ulwick A. Jobs to Be Done: Theory to Practice. USA: Idea Bite Press; 2016

[13] Christensen C, Grossman J, Hwang J. The Innovator's Prescription: A Disruptive Solution for Healthcare. New York: McGraw-Hill; 2009

[14] Von Hippel E. Sources of Innovation. Cambridge: The MIT Press; 1988

[15] Chesbrough H. Open Innovation: The New Imperative for Creating and Profiting from Technology. Cambridge: Harvard Business School Press; 2003

[16] Von Hippel E. Free Innovation. Cambridge: The MIT Press; 2017

[17] Von Hippel E. Democratizing Innovation. Cambridge: The MIT Press; 2005

[18] Drucker P. Innovation and Entrepreneurship: Practice and Principles. New York: Routledge Classics; 1985

[19] Rogers E. Diffusion of Innovation. 5th ed. New York: Free Press; 2004

[20] Bottorff J. Nursing: A practical science of caring. Advances in Nursing Science. 1991;**14**:26-39

[21] World Health Organization. Nursing and Midwifery. [Internet]. 2022. Available from: https://www.who.int/news-room/fact-sheets/detail/nursing-and-midwifery. [Accessed: January 3, 2023]

[22] McDonald L. Florence nightingale and Mary Seacole on nursing and health care. Journal of Advanced Nursing. 2014;**70**:1436-1444. DOI: 10.1111/jan.12291

[23] The Nightingale Society. Florence Nightingale, the founder of modern nursing. [Internet]. 2023. Available from: https://nightingalesociety.com/papers/florence-nightingale-founder-of-modern-nursing/. [Accessed: January 8, 2023]

[24] Fee E, Garofalo ME. Florence nightingale and the Crimean war. American Journal of Public Health. 2010;**100**:1591. DOI: 10.2105/AJPH.2009.188607

[25] Rappaport H. A Historian's Quest to Unravel the Secrets of Mary Seacole, an Innovative Long-Overlooked Black Nurse. [Internet]. 2022. Available from: https://www.smithsonianmag.com/history/a-historians-quest-to-unravel-the-secrets-of-mary-seacole-an-innovative-long-overlooked-black-nurse-180980527/. [Accessed: January 16, 2023]

[26] American Public Health Association. The Definition and Practice of Public Health Nursing. [Internet]. 2013. Available from: https://www.apha.org/media/Files/PDF/membergroups/PHN/NursingDefinition.ashx [Accessed: January 8, 2023]

[27] World Population Review. 2023 World Population by Country [Internet]. 2023. Available from: https://worldpopulationreview.com/. [Accessed: January 7, 2023]

[28] Rothberg E. Lillian Wald. [Internet]. n.d. Available from: https://www.womenshistory.org/education-resources/biographies/lillian-wald. [Accessed: January 8, 2023]

[29] AANP. Loretta C. Ford, Co-founder of Nurse Practitioner (NP) Profession, Receives U.S. Surgeon General's Medallion for Contributions to Nation's Health. [Internet]. 2020. Available from: https://www.aanp.org/news-feed/loretta-c-ford-co-founder-of-nurse-practitioner-np-profession-receives-u-s-surgeon-generals-medallion-for-contributions-to-nations-health. [Accessed: January 16, 2023]

[30] AANP. NP Fact Sheet. [Internet]. 2023. Available from: https://www.aanp.org/about/all-about-nps/np-fact-sheet. [Accessed: January 8, 2023]

[31] The American Red Cross. Clara Barton [Internet]. 2023. Available from: https://www.redcross.org/about-us/who-we-are/history/clarabarton.html# :~:text=Barton%20risked%20her%20life%20to,guided%20her%20throughout%20her%20life. [Accessed: January 8, 2023]

[32] Hiestand W. Think different: Inventions and innovations by nurses, 1850 to 1950. American Journal of Nursing. 2000;**100**:72-77

[33] Weir W. 'Mrs. Chase' is a Medical Marvel [Internet]. 2012. Available from: https://www.courant.com/health/hc-xpm-2012-03-29-hc-mrs-chase-hartford-hospital-0238-20120327-story.html. [Accessed: January 16, 2023]

[34] Hely EG. Sister Elizabeth Kenny: Story of the "Sylvia" Stretcher. [Internet]. 1927. Available from: https://trove.nla.gov.au/newspaper/article/158297457. [Accessed: January 16, 2023]

[35] Kelley T. Identify opportunities to improve the EHR experience. American Journal Nurse Journal. 2022;**17**. DOI: 10.51256/AJN122233. Available from: https://www.myamericannurse.com/identify-opportunities-to-improve-the-ehr-experience/

[36] Office of the National Coordinator for Health Information Technology. Adoption of Electronic Health Records by Hospital Service Type 2019-2021. Health IT Quick Stat #60 [Internet]. 2022. Available from: healthit.gov/data/quickstats/adoption-electronic-health-records-hospital-service-type-2019-2021 [Accessed: January 3, 2023]

[37] Office of the National Coordinator for Health Information Technology. Office-Based Physician Electronic Health Record Adoption. Health IT Quick Stat #50 [Internet]. n.d. Available from: healthit.gov/data/quickstats/office-based-physician-electronic-health-record-adoption. [Accessed: January 3, 2023]

[38] Kelley T. Electronic Health Records for Quality Nursing and Health Care. Lancaster: Destech Publications; 2016

[39] Institute of Medicine. Crossing the Quality Chasm. Washington: National Academy Press; 2001

[40] Agency for Healthcare Quality. Understanding Quality Measurement. [Internet]. 2020. Available from: https://www.ahrq.gov/patient-safety/quality-resources/tools/chtoolbx/understand/index.html#:~:text=The%20Institute%20of%20Medicine%20defines,consistent%20with%20current%20professional%20knowledge.%22 [Accessed: January 7, 2023]

[41] Kelley T, Docherty S, Brandon D. Information needed to support knowing the patient. Advances in Nursing Science. 2013;**36**:351-363. DOI: 10.1097/ANS.0000000000000006

[42] Design Thinking for Health [Internet]. 2022. Available from: https://designthinkingforhealth.org/#:~:text=Design %20Thinking%20is%20a%20framework,re%20in%20the%20right%20place! [Accessed: January 7, 2023]

[43] Centers for Disease Control and Prevention. Facts about Falls [Internet]. 2021. Available from: https://www.cdc.gov/falls/facts.html#:~:text=each%20year%2C%203%20million%20older,emergency%20departments%20for%20fall%20injuries.&text=Over%20800%2C000%20patients%20a%20year,head%20injury%20or%20hip%20fracture [Accessed: January 3, 2023]

[44] Khalifa M, Khalid P. Reducing unnecessary laboratory testing using health informatics applications: A case study on a tertiary care hospital. Procedia Computer Science. 2014;**37**:253-260

[45] Weberg D, Davidson S. Leadership for Evidence-Based Innovation in Nursing and Health Professions. 2nd ed. Burlington: Jones and Bartlett Learning; 2019

[46] Morris ZS, Wooding S, Grant J. The answer is 17 years, what is the question: Understanding time lags in translational research. Journal of the Royal Society of Medicine. 2011;**104**:510-520. DOI: 10.1258/jrsm.2011.110180

[47] Healthy People 2030. Social Determinants of Health [Internet]. n.d. Available from: https://health.gov/healthypeople/priority-areas/social-determinants-health. [Accessed: January 16, 2023]

[48] Kelley T. What does it mean to be a nurse innovator? [Internet]. 2021. Available from: https://www.kevinmd.com/2021/11/what-does-it-mean-to-be-a-nurse-innovator.html#:~:text=A%20nurse%20innovator%20is%20a,products%2C%20

processes%2C%20and%20services [Accessed: January 16, 2023]

[49] Boyer EL. Scholarship Reconsidered: Priorities of the Professoriate. Carnegie Foundation of the Advancement of Teaching: Princeton; 1990

[50] Centers for Medicare and Medicaid Services. CMS Roadmaps Overview. [Internet]. n.d. Available from: https://www.cms.gov/medicare/quality-initiatives-patient-assessment-instruments/qualityinitiativesgeninfo/downloads/roadmapoverview_oea_1-16.pdf [Accessed: January 16, 2023]

[51] CMS.gov. Medicare Telemedicine Health Care Provider Fact Sheet. [Internet]. 2020. Available from: https://www.cms.gov/newsroom/fact-sheets/medicare-telemedicine-health-care-provider-fact-sheet. [Accessed: January 16, 2023]

[52] Hyder MA, Razzak J. Telemedicine in the United States: An introduction for students and residents. Journal of Medical Internet Research. 2020;**22**:e20839

[53] World Health Organization. Health Innovation for Impact. [Internet]. 2023. Available from https://www.who.int/teams/digital-health-and-innovation/health-innovation-for-impact. [Accessed: January 7, 2023]

[54] ANA Enterprise. Innovation. [Internet]. n.d. Available from: https://www.nursingworld.org/practice-policy/innovation [Accessed: January 8, 2023]

[55] American Association of Colleges of Nursing. The Re-envisioned Essentials: Infusing Innovation in Academic Nursing. [Internet]. 2021. Available from: https://www.aacnnursing.org/Professional-Development/WebinarInfo/sessionaltcd/WF21_09_16. [Accessed: January 8, 2023]

Chapter 2

Adaptive Web-Based Technology Aiming at Improving Learning of Medication Calculation Skills for Nursing Students

Monika Ravik and Kristoffer Ravik Andresen

Abstract

Medication calculation skills are in great demand among registered nurses. However, miscalculations are a common medication error performed by registered nurses in the clinical setting. Medication calculation errors are common causes of unintended harm to patients of all ages. Mastery of medication calculation skills is one of the tasks nursing students should achieve during their education. Outcome measures, however, indicate that for many students, accurate medication calculations are challenging to both learn and master. This justifies the need for effective learning and teaching approaches in medication calculation skills for nursing students. In recent years, interactive and dynamic learning resources in the form of technological devices and interventions have been developed and implemented to improve nursing students' learning opportunities in medication calculation skills. Research suggests that web-based technologies can enhance learning opportunities in medication calculations. However, for students who have inadequate knowledge, opportunities, and abilities in learning, progression slows down, and more time must be spent on learning. Adaptive web-based learning technology is an emerging technology that have additional learning benefits than traditional interactive web-based learning technologies. This chapter describes the potential of adaptive web-based learning technologies to support learning of medication calculation skills.

Keywords: web-based learning, interactive learning, adaptive web-based learning, medication calculation skills, health care education, health care students, medication calculations, medication calculation skills

1. Introduction

1.1 Learning and development of professional competence in medication calculation skills

Professional competence is considered as an essential ingredient to provide effective nursing care and to ensure patient safety [1, 2]. Professional competence is

IntechOpen

defined as the ability to use a set of knowledge, skills, attitudes, clinical reasoning, and behaviors to successfully perform jobs, roles, or responsibilities [3]. Medication calculation skills are in great demand among registered nurses [4]. To provide high-quality and safe care to patients, registered nurses need to be competent in medication calculations [5]. However, miscalculations are a common medication error performed by registered nurses in the clinical setting [5–7]. Medication calculation errors are common causes of unintended harm, such as injury and death, to patients of all ages [7, 8]. Miscalculations also affect patients' length of stay and the financial cost of healthcare services [9]. Miscalculations have to be avoided to protect patients against undesirable consequences such as injury and death [9, 10].

Nursing students go through extensive education, in both the academic and the clinical setting, to develop professional competence so that they are prepared to meet the patients' needs and to provide care with high quality [11, 12]. Mastery of medication calculation skills is one of the tasks nursing students should achieve during their education [12]. Outcome measures, however, indicate that for many students, accurate medication calculations are challenging to both learn and master [13–15]. For example, in a European study including six countries, the authors found that even simple calculation tasks were challenging to master correctly for nursing students [15]. Medication calculation skills should be acknowledged as a well-defined competency in nursing education curricula and continuing education programs [6, 12, 16].

Improving the medication calculation skills of nursing students has been an ongoing challenge for nursing educators [9, 15, 17]. The issue lies in designing pedagogical, monitoring, and tutoring scenarios to support students to learn medication calculation skills appropriately [13, 17]. Currently, there are several global educational initiatives to enhance learning and thereby prevent medication calculation errors. Most common are textbooks that aim to provide students with theoretical and practical knowledge in calculation skills [18]. Other resources that have been developed to facilitate student learning include audio files, pictures, animations, simulations, workshops, blended learning, and simple tests [19–22]. In an attempt to respond to the demands of patient safety, many web-based learning resources have also been developed over several years to assist students and professionals in the learning of medication calculations [23–30].

1.1.1 Web-based learning

Web-based learning is increasing from the extensively available and easily accessible connection to the Web [31, 32]. In web-based learning, a computer, such as for example a laptop or mobile phone, is used for instructional processes and is a key component of the educational intervention [33]. Web-based learning allows students to acquire knowledge in risk-free environments without involving real patients, in addition to allowing the learning intervention to be used at a time and place convenient for the students [32, 34]. This means that students can access web-based learning in real time or according to their own schedules, meaning a synchronous and an asynchronous approach to learning. Such flexibility is reported to be a core benefit with web-based learning [34, 35].

Web-based learning that only is based on a network of static hypertext pages provides students with passive and inadequate learning experiences [33]. However, in the recent years of web-based development, several web-based learning developers have implemented different kinds of interactive web-based learning interventions, providing students with opportunities to make their own choices from the various options available based on their understanding of a task or situation [17, 32]. In this lens, students are given a hands-on approach to web-based learning, working with questions or quizzes and assessment activities when learning a task. This active learning approach engages students with the learning material [34]. Students are required to participate in the learning process actively, rather than simply be passive receivers of information [35].

Since the advent of web-based learning, various web-based learning resources have been developed to improve learning in medication calculation skills [23, 24, 27, 36–38]. However, technological learning interventions do not necessarily provide benefits in medication calculation skills for all students. Kim and Park [27], for example, studied the effectiveness of an interactive smartphone-based dosage calculation training app in a Korean context and revealed that the app improved nursing students' calculation skills but only for students with higher prior knowledge. The smartphone-based training program had an inadequate effect on knowledge building in students with lower prior knowledge. In a Norwegian context, Foss et al. [24] developed the interactive web-based learning resource 'The Medication Game.' Nursing students experienced the web-based learning resource to be fun to use, but the authors concluded that the learning resource did not significantly improve the students' test results in medication calculations. Both students and professionals continue to struggle with the learning and mastering of medication calculation skills [5, 6, 13, 26, 27]. This brings to the fact that even interactive web-based learning resources do not ensure learning and competence development in medication calculations for all learners.

Students progress at different paces; while some individuals learn fast, others learn more slowly [27]. It is imperative to design and develop web-based learning resources that provide appropriate learning opportunities in medication calculation skills for meeting knowledge requirements of all learners [15, 27]. The learning of medication calculation skills should be based on the individual student's learning needs and abilities in learning, an *adaptive approach* to learning, and not in a system that 'fits all' [39]. By adaptive technology, we mean an algorithm that can determine what knowledge the individual student lacks, what kind of feedback the individual student needs, and what challenges the student should face [40–42].

1.1.2 Adaptive web-based learning

Adaptive means adaptation, and adaptive learning is the same as adapted training. Adaptive learning is an educational method that uses web-based learning resources to specially adapt learning materials and assignments to the individual's prior knowledge and skill level [40–43]. In adaptive web-based learning, the software observes one or more aspects of learning, most often whether if the student has answered correctly or has errors in tasks, and then analyzes the observations in order to personalize the learning materials offered by the web-based learning resource [41, 42]. This means that the software does an analysis of what the student has mastered and not and the need the individual has for learning to achieve progression in their understanding and mastery. In such an approach to learning, the adaptive web-based learning resource will help a student obtain information in a form that fits the individual's characteristics and fulfills the student's real learning needs automatically, as well as help the student to avoid the challenges of information overload [40–42]. Many students do not understand themselves as learners in order to understand their learning needs and abilities in learning [44]. Consequently, students do not understand their strength and limitations, making it challenging for students to select what tasks they need to learn and practice. Moreover, they make inappropriate choices in both learning objectives and approaches to studying, for example, surface and deep approaches to studying and learning [45].

Development of adaptive web-based learning resources in the field of healthcare education is in its infancy [39, 40, 43, 46]. Fontaine et al. [40] have conducted a systematic review including 21 articles, enrolling 3684 health professionals and students. Clinical topics were in particular related to diagnostic testing, and no studies were related to medication calculation skills. In a recent scoping literature review by Andersen et al. [43], aiming to explore characteristics with adaptive learning technologies blended into nursing education, none of the six studies included in the review concerned medication calculation skills. Andresen [39] has in a Norwegian context developed an adaptive web-based learning resource related to medication calculation skills, and the learning resource is revised and adjusted until June 2022. This emerging web-based learning resource could hold promise for enhanced learning and development of competence in medication calculation skills. It is challenging to develop a web-based learning resource combining pedagogical rules with adaptive web-based technology in order to give students more personalized learning experiences [42, 47]. First, we describe the emerging web-based learning resource, and then, we suggest how the web-based learning resource can contribute to learning. Following this, we define research to be conducted to evaluate and test the adaptive web-based learning resource.

2. Description of emerging technology, an adaptive web-based learning resource

A big challenge in developing an educational web-based learning resource is the intelligent and personalized resource recommendation for learners, how to implement personalized facilities by understanding the learner's personal characteristics such as learning needs and abilities in learning [42, 47]. The adaptive web-based learning resource designed by Andresen [39] provides a personalized approach to learning of medication calculation skills, implying the individual student's level of calculations to be considered.

A key point was the use of the Technological, Pedagogical, and Content Knowledge (TPACK) model [48] (**Figure 1**) to design and develop the adaptive technological learning resource for medication calculations. Such knowledge is important to possess in order to realize the potential benefits from the web-based learning technology [43, 48]. Using the TPACK model contributed to a learning resource, shifting the accent from simple information transmission to a constructivist way of learning [46].

Figure 1 illustrates that the TPACK model consists of three types of knowledge (technological, pedagogical, and content knowledge) and further that the TPACK model's three types of knowledge are mutually dependent for innovative teaching and learning. By differentiating among these types of knowledge, the TPACK model outlines how content and pedagogy form the foundation of effective education, while the technology used should communicate the content and support the pedagogy to enhance students' learning experience. **Content knowledge** is domain-specific knowledge and, in this case, related to medication calculations, for example, what formulas (dose–quantity–strength) to be used when calculating medicines in different categories (tablets, injections, drops etc.).

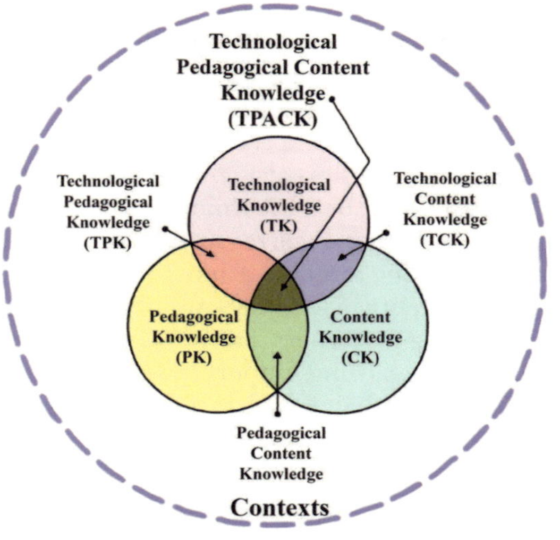

Figure 1.
The TPACK model [48].

Pedagogical knowledge describes theoretical learning approaches, lesson planning, and assessments. The adaptive web-based learning technology in medication calculations is proposed as a person-centered long-term strategy for learning and developing essential medication calculation skills. A cognitive perspective on learning is underpinned by the idea that individual learning is a result of a re-construction of knowledge, implying that new knowledge builds on previous knowledge [49]. The adaptive web-based learning resource was also developed based on the theoretical understanding of scaffolding, a process in which a more knowledgeable 'other' demonstrates how to perform a specific task, then allows the learner to work independently, offering support as needed [50]. Vygotsky [50] related this to the zone of proximal development (ZPD), which describes the difference between what a learner can do independently and what he/she can do with support or guidance from the more knowledgeable 'other.' The adaptive web-based learning technology is the more knowledgeable 'other,' supporting the learner to be in a flow zone, which is the balance between what is too challenging and what is too easy to be mastered independently. In such a way, learning is adapted to the individual student's learning needs and abilities in learning. Students will be kept continuously motivated for learning and development when a computer guides them into their personal flow zone [43]. Additionally, the learning and teaching principle 'constructive alignment' has been taken into consideration, as learning goals, learning activities, and assessment methods have been appropriately aligned [51]. The adaptive web-based learning resource was developed in line with these theoretical approaches, as it is based on how students learn and develop knowledge in order to achieve understanding and competence. Theoretical approaches are commonly applied to inform development of web-based learning resources [46].

Technological knowledge concerns understanding the function of a web-based learning resource and exploring its possibilities for assisting or impeding learning in a specific subject area [48]. Adaptivity is implemented into the web-based learning resource via content adaption and link adaption: the former is how the learning outcomes/tasks are presented, and the latter is how the student navigates between the content adaption [40, 47]. In this way, the student is provided with feedback and assessments that are the most appropriate for the student's medication calculation level, learning needs, and abilities in learning [41].

In summary, the TPACK model is implemented into the adaptive web-based learning resource via content and link adaption. The student's medication calculation level anticipates the types of medication calculations and learning support (content knowledge) that best address the student's learning needs and thereby increase learning efficacy. The student's correct and incorrect medication calculations are stored in the adaptive web-based learning resource to build the individual student's profile (knowledge, learning needs, ability in learning) and thereby adapt the presentation of education material according to learners' profile. In this way, computer algorithms coordinate the interactions and learning support to address the content, knowledge, learning needs, and ability in learning of each individual student in medication calculations (technological knowledge). Students are given opportunities to engage in repetitive learning and further be engaged in less challenging medication calculations before being engaged in more challenging medication calculations, which highlights the learning of medication calculation skills as a developmental trajectory (pedagogical knowledge). The adaptive web-based learning resource is in line with a complex learning resource, providing meaningful and constructive feedback around learning and motivating and stimulating reflection within the learning situation [52].

2.1 Reflections and expectations of the adaptive web-based learning resource in medication calculations

To ensure that nursing students are competent in medication calculation skills, nursing education must bear the responsibility for the development and implementation of pedagogical strategies for teaching, learning, and assessing medication calculations [15]. Including any web-based learning resources does not necessarily guarantee better learning outcomes in medication calculation skills [27]. Students may fail to effectively grasp important information and learning opportunities due to having total freedom in browsing the web-based learning objectives/tasks. Self-directed learning (known as learning independently) can be challenging even in higher education, even for the brightest and most motivated students [53]. The fact that students can decide which tasks they want to learn and what tasks to solve by quizzes is not to be understood as being adaptive but only an interactive non-adaptive function that stimulates an active approach to learning [40, 41].

We suggest that an adaptive web-based learning resource will facilitate acquisition of medication calculation skills so that students become competent in medication calculations. An adaptive web-based learning resource will enable students to learn more comprehensively through independent learning with individual accountability and mastery of learning [40, 42]. The existing literature is limited to the development of web-based learning resources in medication calculations without taking into consideration the individual's learning needs and abilities in learning. The adaptive web-based learning resource developed by Andresen (2018), however, tailors learning to each individual student instead of providing the same traditional educational material to all students in a one-size-fits-all model. The adaptive element of the web-based learning resource is considered to be a person-centered approach to learning, by providing students with personalized learning even in a large group or clinical setting and thus avoiding cognitive overload [49] when learning medication calculations. Furthermore, students are enabled to be active and engaged learners, with individualized feedback based on their ZPD [50], important for optimal learning and development of their medication calculation skills.

The adaptive web-based learning resource is expected to allow educators teaching medication calculation skills to monitor nursing students' learning processes, to determine which aspects of medication calculation skills students find easy or difficult to master, and, in such a lens, to identify common challenges suitable for whole-class teaching. In this way, the adaptive web-based learning resource will function as a formative assessment resource to guide teachers as to what they should focus on when teaching in a group. In such an approach to teaching and learning in medication calculations, students' learning will become more visible and useful, to both teachers and nursing students. Teachers need to be aware of students' learning and development of knowledge to provide appropriate learning experiences for students [54]. Moreover, the adaptive web-based learning resource is assumed to be transferable to other healthcare professionals, for example, students in social work, paramedics, and medicine, who also are reported to have challenges in learning and developing knowledge and competence in medication calculation skills [55–57].

3. Conclusion

This chapter has proposed an adaptive recommendation approach of educational resources in learning medication calculation skills in nursing education. The aim of this recommendation was to provide better learning opportunities in medication calculations for students according to the individual student's learning needs and abilities in learning. We have shown how to combine pedagogical rules with an adaptive web-based learning resource in order to give students more personalized learning experiences. We believe that nursing students will appropriately learn and develop medication calculation skills that are necessary to practice proper and safe nursing when they engage in using the adaptive web-based learning resource. How web-based learning resources are shaping learning in higher education is, however, less explored [42]. Due to the promising benefits of adaptive web-based learning [39, 42], we argue that directions for future research should be guided by the voices of the learners who will use the adaptive web-based learning resource when learning and developing medication calculation skills.

This complex adaptive web-based learning resource needs to be evaluated and tested to obtain knowledge of the consequences of implementing the resource in terms of its benefits and drawbacks in areas such as learning outcomes, learning experiences, user friendliness, motivation for learning outside the classroom, lightening the burden on the teaching staff when instructing large numbers of students, improved patient safety due to less miscalculations, and cost effectiveness due to accurate calculations in the clinical setting. Kabudi et al. [42] have emphasized the importance of evaluating adaptive web-based learning resources, because they can offer significant benefit for the individual learner.

Funding

This book chapter did not receive any specific grant from funding agencies in the public, commercial, or not-for-profit sectors.

Availability of data and materials

Given the nature of this work, there is no dataset used and/or analyzed.

Author details

Monika Ravik[1*] and Kristoffer Ravik Andresen[2]

1 Faculty of Health and Social Studies, University of South-Eastern Norway, Porsgrunn, Norway

2 Self-Employed (Software Developer), Hunsrødskogen, Sandefjord, Norway

*Address all correspondence to: monika.ravik@usn.no

References

[1] Fukada M. Nursing competency: Definition, structure and development. Yonago. Acta Medica. 2018;**61**:1-7

[2] Kieft RA, de Brouwer BB, Francke AL, et al. How nurses and their work environment affect patient experiences of the quality of care: A qualitative study. BMC Health Services Research. 2014;**14**:1-10

[3] Cowan DT, Norman I, Coopamah VP. Competence in nursing practice: A controversial concept - a focused review of literature. Accident and Emergency Nursing. 2007;**15**:20-26

[4] Härkänen M, Luokkamäki S, Saano S, et al. Identifying risk areas of medication administration process for developing an interactive three-dimensional game intervention. Computers, Informatics, Nursing. 2020;**38**:524-533

[5] Luokkamäki S, Härkänen M, Saano S, et al. Registered nurses' medication administration skills: A systematic review. Scandinavian Journal of Caring Sciences. 2020;**35**:37-54

[6] Awajeh AM, Issa MR, Abuelian A, et al. An evaluation of the drug calculation skills of registered nurses in the critical Care Department at a Tertiary Hospital in KSA. Journal of Nursing and Health Studies. 2019;**4**:1-4

[7] Mulac A, Taxis K, Hagesaether E, et al. Severe and fatal medication errors in hospitals: Findings from the Norwegian incident reporting system. European Journal of Hospital Pharmacy. 2020;**0**:1-6

[8] Alsaidan J, Portlock J, Aljadhey HS, et al. Systematic review of the safety of medication use in inpatient, outpatient and primary care settings in the Gulf cooperation council countries. Saudi Pharmaceutical Journal. 2018;**26**:977-1011

[9] WHO. The third WHO Global Patient Safety Challenge: Medication Without Harm. The third WHO Global Patient Safety Challenge: Medication Without Harm. 2017. Available from: https://www.who.int/patientsafety/medication-safety/en

[10] Björkstén KS, Bergqvist M, Andersén-Karlsson E, et al. Medication errors as malpractice-a qualitative content analysis of 585 medication errors by nurses in Sweden. BMC Health Services Research. 2016;**16**:1-8

[11] Bagnasco A, Galaverna L, Aleo G, et al. Mathematical calculation skills required for drug administration in undergraduate nursing students to ensure patient safety: A descriptive study. Nurse Education in Practice. 2016;**16**:33-39

[12] Lazare M-B. The lived experiences of undergraduate nursing students learning drug dosage calculation. International Journal of Nursing Clinical Practices. 2018;**5**:1-13

[13] Caboral-Stevens M, Ignacio R, Newberry G. Undergraduate nursing students' pharmacology knowledge and risk error estimate. Nurse Education Today. 2020;**93**:1-6

[14] Castaldo A, Ferrentino M, Ferrario E, et al. Factors contributing to medication errors: A descriptive qualitative study of Italian nursing students. Nurse Education Today. 2022;**118**:1-7

[15] Elonen I, Salminen L, Brasaitė-Abromė I, et al. Medication calculation skills of graduating nursing students

within European context. Journal of Clinical Nursing. 2021;**31**:548-558

[16] Fleming S, Brady A-M, Malone A-M. An evaluation of the drug calculation skills of registered nurses. Nurse Education in Practice. 2014;**14**:55-61

[17] Jarvis DH, McCullough KD, McParland TR. Nurse education and mathematical competency: Implementation of an online, self-directed, prerequisite model. IJERPH. 2021;**18**:1-19

[18] Gatford J, Philips N. Nursing Calculations. 9th ed. Elsevier; 15 Jul 2016. Imprint: Churchill Livingstone. ISBN: 9780702065019

[19] Lee SE, Quinn BL. Incorporating medication administration safety in undergraduate nursing education: A literature review. Nurse Education Today. 2019;**72**:77-83

[20] Stolic S. Educational strategies aimed at improving student nurse's medication calculation skills: A review of the research literature. Nurse Education in Practice. 2014;**14**:491-503

[21] Gill M, Andersen E, Hilsmann N. Best practices for teaching pharmacology to undergraduate nursing students: A systematic review of the literature. Nurse Education Today. 2019;**74**:15-24

[22] Ramjan LM, Stewart L, Salamonson Y, et al. Identifying strategies to assist final semester nursing students to develop numeracy skills: A mixed methods study. Nurse Education Today. 2014;**34**:405-412

[23] Aydin AK, Dinç L. Effects of web-based instruction on nursing Students' arithmetical and drug dosage calculation skills. Computers, Informatics, Nursing. 2017;**35**:262-269

[24] Foss B, Løkken A, Leland A, et al. Digital game-based learning: A supplement for medication calculation drills in nurse education. E-Learning and Digital Media. 2013;**11**:342-349

[25] Mcqueen DS, Begg MJ, Maxwell SRJ. eDrugCalc: An online self-assessment package to enhance medical students' drug dose calculation skills. British Journal of Clinical Pharmacology. 2010;**70**:492-499

[26] Özyazıcıoğlu N, Aydın Aİ, Sürenler S, et al. Evaluation of students' knowledge about paediatric dosage calculations. Nurse Education in Practice. 2018;**28**:34-39

[27] Park KY, Kim MS. Outcomes of a drug dosage calculation training smartphone app on learning achievement, metacognition, and flow state according to prior knowledge. Eurasia Journal of Mathematics, Science and Technology. 2018;**14**:2867-2876

[28] Pourteimour S, Hemmati Malsak Pak M, Jasemi M, et al. The effect of smartphone-based application learning on the nursing students' performance in preventing medication errors in the pediatric units. Pediatric Quality and Safety. 2019;**4**:1-7

[29] Simonsen BO, Daehlin GK, Johansson I, et al. Improvement of drug dose calculations by classroom teaching or e-learning: A randomised controlled trial in nurses. BMJ Open. 2014;**4**:1-9

[30] Van Lancker A, Baldewijns K, Verhaeghe R, et al. The effectiveness of an e-learning course on medication calculation in nursing students: A clustered quasi-experimental study. Journal of Advanced Nursing. 2016;**72**:2054-2064

[31] Dunleavy G, Nikolaou CK, Nifakos S, et al. Mobile digital education for health professions: Systematic review and

meta-analysis by the digital health education collaboration. Journal of Medical Internet Research. 2019;**21**:1-17

[32] Qurat-ul-Ain Q-A, Shahid F, Aleem M, et al. A review of technological tools in teaching and learning computer science. Eurasia Journal of Mathematics, Science and Technology. 2019;**15**:1-17

[33] Alharthi AD, Spichkova M, Hamilton M. Sustainability requirements for eLearning systems: A systematic literature review and analysis. Requirements Engineering. 2019;**24**:523-543

[34] Regmi K, Jones L. A systematic review of the factors – Enablers and barriers – Affecting e-learning in health sciences education. BMC Medical Education. 2020;**20**:91

[35] Webb L, Clough J, O'Reilly D, et al. The utility and impact of information communication technology (ICT) for pre-registration nurse education: A narrative synthesis systematic review. Nurse Education Today. 2017;**48**:160-171

[36] Bull ER, Mason C, Junior FD, et al. Developing nurse medication safety training in a health partnership in Mozambique using behavioural science. Globalization and Health. 2017;**13**:45

[37] Mettiäinen S, Luojus K, Salminen S, et al. Web course on medication administration strengthens nursing students' competence prior to graduation. Nurse Education in Practice. 2014;**14**:368-373

[38] Renmarker E, Carlson E. Evaluation of Swedish nursing students' experience of a web-based platform for drug calculation. Nurse Education in Practice. 2019;**38**:89-95

[39] Andresen K. Development and Exploration of an Adaptive Learning System in Medication Calculation in Nursing [Thesis]. Norway: Norwegian University of Science and Technology (NTNU); 2018

[40] Fontaine G, Cossette S, Maheu-Cadotte M-A, et al. Efficacy of adaptive e-learning for health professionals and students: A systematic review and meta-analysis. BMJ Open. 2019;**9**:1-17

[41] Jagust T, Boticki I. Mobile learning system for enabling collaborative and adaptive pedagogies with modular digital learning contents. Journal of Computer Education. 2019;**6**:335-362

[42] Kabudi T, Pappas I, Olsen DH. AI-enabled adaptive learning systems: A systematic mapping of the literature. Computers and Education: Artificial Intelligence. 2021;**2**:1-12

[43] Andersen BL, Jørnø RL, Nortvig A-M. Blending adaptive learning technology into nursing education: A scoping review. Contemporary Educational Technology. 2022;**14**:1-11

[44] Lodge JM, Kennedy G, Lockyer L, et al. Understanding difficulties and resulting confusion in learning: An integrative review. Frontiers in Education. 2018;**3**:1-10

[45] Marton F, Säljö R. On qualitative differences in learning. I - outcome and process. British Journal of Educational Psychology. 1976;**46**:4-11

[46] O'Connor S, Kennedy S, Wang Y, et al. Theories informing technology enhanced learning in nursing and midwifery education: A systematic review and typological classification. Nurse Education Today. 2022;**118**:1-11

[47] Shershneva V, Vainshtein Y, Kochetkova T, et al. Technological approach to development of adaptive

e-learning system. SHS Web of Conferences. 2019;**66**:01014

[48] Koehler MJ, Mishra P. What is technological pedagogical content knowledge? CITE. 2009;**9**:60-70

[49] Piaget J. The Equilibration of Cognitive Structures. The Central Problem of Intellectual Development. Chicago: University of Chicago Press; 1985

[50] Vygotsky LS. Mind in Society: The Development of Higher Psychological Processes. Cambridge, Mass: Harvard University Press; 1978

[51] Biggs J. Student Approaches to Learning and Studying. Hawthorn, Victoria: Australian Council for Educational Research; 1987

[52] Lillejord S, Børte K, Nesje K, et al. Learning and Teaching with Technology in Higher Education – A Systematic Review. Oslo: Knowledge center for Education; 2018

[53] Abdou H, Sleem W, EL-Wkeel N. Nursing students readiness and perspective toward self-directed learning. Mansoura Nursing Journal. 2021;**8**:77-90

[54] Hattie J. The applicability of visible learning to higher education. Scholarship of Teaching and Learning in Psychology. 2015;**1**:79-91

[55] Geoghegan SE, Clarke E, Byrne D, et al. Preparedness of newly qualified doctors in Ireland for prescribing in clinical practice: Preparedness of newly qualified doctors in Ireland for prescribing. British Journal of Clinical Pharmacology. 2017;**83**:1826-1834

[56] Boyle MJ. Drug calculation ability of qualified paramedics: A pilot study. World Journal of Emergency Medicine. 2018;**9**:41-45

[57] Lee MCR, Tully MP, et al. Readiness to prescribe: Using educational design to untie the Gordian knot. PLoS One. 2020;**15**:1-12

Chapter 3

Telenursing Future in Solving the Nursing Global Workforce Gap

Zainab Attia Abdallah, Engy Abdel Rahman Khamis, Fatma M. Ibrahim and Ayiat Allah Wagdy Farag

Abstract

Although there are 28 million nurses worldwide, it is not enough to meet patient needs. So we face a future with too much work, with too few workers. Telenursing can help in solving this issue by utilizing the technology in providing distance healthcare and health education to patients/clients with lower costs, effective services and proper clients' satisfaction especially in rural areas through insufficient accessibility to local clinics or hospitals. Telenursing can use phone calls, video visits and remote monitoring devices in different nursing fields as family, pediatric, geriatric nursing and/or others. Telenursing can improve the quality of nursing care for patients by building relationships with them and improve the preferable outcomes. Telenursing also can decrease the work burden on nurses and direct contacts with patients with negative related health consequences specially after COVID 19 pandemic.

Keywords: telenursing, telehealth, telemedicine, distance healthcare, nursing practice, nursing education, nursing shortage, technology, COVID 19 pandemic

1. Introduction

Telenursing means use of digital devices as phone calls, video visits and remote monitoring devices in different nursing fields as family, pediatric, geriatric nursing and/or others. Telenursing means as the nursing services can be provided through electronic platforms, which includes phone calls, video conferences and remote patients' monitoring through different electronic devices. Applying of telenursing in healthcare systems with related health and safety benefits, can provide high quality of life and significant financial benefits to all of patients, family and health and welfare services. It creates the necessary for the development of electronic learning (e-learning) in nursing, telenursing simulation, evidence based nursing practice and nursing research. Telenursing also includes health education services, vital signs' regular remote monitoring, ECG or blood pressure and remote doctor or nurse-patient consultations as needed [1].

According to the American Telemedicine Association, 50% of health services could be provided by telehealth. To cover the needs of healthcare systems and to achieve the balance between the health team workforce and the quality of care, we need to 1.1 million new registered nurses at least. The Global Healthcare Expert, Dr. Mark Britnell, reported that by 2030, the global will face a future with too much work, with too few workers. He said: "We will reach 18 million health workers short by 2030 and this represents a gap to care." So, the need for solving the nursing and health team workforce become very necessary from now. Appearance of many global technological methods in health care delivery systems through COVID 19 pandemic, may make the problem solution slightly easy [2].

Telehealth offers flexibility and accessibility of patients to their documents and nurses and health care providers safely from home, with more control of their health care. Additionally, nurses can be accessed with telehealth equipment to host virtual meetings with their patients. Using telenursing in providing health care has several advantages as cost savings, convenience, and overcoming patients' care with mobility limitations especially rural areas' citizens who meet difficulties in accessibility to healthcare resources [3].

The integration of telenursing principles in academic programs becomes very necessary to expand the documentation bases for telenursing services and to develop such a new nursing theory involving the impact of telenursing on patient, family, community, health care delivery systems and research protocols. The future challenges in telenursing could be the technological advancement in health care systems and the training of future nurses and health care providers based on clinical simulation and online courses to apply distance-based nursing care [4].

2. Overview of telehealth and telenursing

Telehealth or telemedicine is defined as where a health provider can provide care or health services without a direct face-to-face office visit, but from a distance and is done electronically, online with internet access with different devices as a computer, tablet or smartphone. Telemedicine also has many other definitions as Mobile Health or Health Mobile, Telehealth and E-Health. Telehealth Nursing is applying of different telehealth technologies as tools to provide health care in a variety of ways as addressing of social determinants of health such as [5]:

- Access for vulnerable patients and older populations.
- Greater access for rural areas.
- Patients with multiple chronic illnesses with difficulty travel.
- Patient education.
- Remote patient monitoring.

Telenursing refers to using of information technology in providing nursing care and services through mobile devices and computers whenever distance exists between patient-nurse, or between a number of nurses or health care providers. Based on accessibility of mobile devices, telehealth becomes more prevalent as one of healthcare options. Telenursing as a field, is a part of telemedicine, and has a direct and indirect contacts with other medical applications and others of non-medical, as tele-diagnosis, teleconsultation and tele-monitoring. Telenursing enables patients from connecting nurses through mobile devices/applications, video technology, computers and also remote patient monitoring. So healthcare does not be limited to in-patient clinical setting, patient can access nurse and/or primary care providers at any location [6].

There is a variety of tools using in providing health care through telenursing. As well as, nurses can use telenursing for sending information to patients through websites or mobile applications. They can monitor patient condition regularly through remote monitoring. However, telehealth and telenursing are not comprehensive enough and still being developed, they become more utilized than ever as clients are preferring face to face interaction with nurses or other healthcare providers. Recently, telenursing is growing up in many countries. This growing in some countries may be because of the preoccupation in driving down the affordability of health care services, increasing of aging and chronically ill persons and the increase in desiring of coverage of health care to distant, rural areas, small/sparsely populated regions. There are many examples of applying telenursing technology as a tool of providing care as the following [7]:

- Patient education and/or remote patient monitoring.
- Primary care, health promotion, assessment, diagnosis, treatment of and care providing for quarantined patients.
- Tele-nurses or other telehealth provides support and assist providers in remote areas.
- Telenursing in applying school health care.
- Telenursing to prevent and eliminate of direct exposure during epidemics and pandemics such as COVID-19.

3. Historical background of telehealth and telenursing

In 1870s, Graham Bell the inventor of telephone carried out the first telephonic call aiming for management of battery acid burns. In 1912, Australian Inland Mission applied nursing care for nurses in remote areas. In 1929, The first telenursing service was through the Trager pedal radio processing services communication between outpost nurses and flying doctors. In 1960 National Aeronautics and Space Administration (NASA) invented and applied a telemedicine to monitor astronauts' health. During 1970s, some health organizations used nurses to give advices through telephone. In 1974, Mary Quinn documented the Logan airport care providing to patients from Boston through telemedicine [5]. In 1997, the Indian Apollo group of hospitals carried out telemedicine via the first outreach use of communication technology. Following that in 2003, a telehealth certificated course was started by Apollo group of hospitals with cooperation with Annamalai University by training of 30 students in each batch. In 2005, International Council for Nurses (ICN) conducted the international telenursing survey which revealed that nearly 719 tele-nurses responded positively. After 2005 and all over the world, telenursing became to be applied more, and nurses and patients' tele-interaction become more noticed and advanced gradually [8]. By spreading of COVID 19 pandemic in the end of 2019, different countries have directed to use innovative methods for fighting against COVID 19 virus. The main challenges for all healthcare systems all over the world were large number of patients, in addition to who could be cared at home, shortage of health team members especially doctors and nurses, lack of intensive care units' facilities and lack of hospital capacities. Therefore, recent methods had been proposed, tele-nursing was one of the good ways to control COVID 19 pandemic [9].

4. Telenursing' legal, ethical and regulatory issues

Telenursing is surrounded by legal, ethical and many regulatory issues, as what happens with telehealth. Those legal issues such as malpractice, negligence and accountability, etc. are also still repeated and difficult to address. Ethical issues also include maintaining autonomy, patient's integrity as well as harmless of clients. In many countries, practical telenursing is forbidden because, the tele-nurse must have a doubled license; one in state/country of residence and another in the location where patient receiving telecare and services. So, the *telenursing licensure* helps in resolving some of these issues [10].

Telenursing professionals store and chart patient data using an electronic medical record (EMR). Transmission of digital clinical data can increase the risk that outside sources may break the confidentiality of sensitive patient information by intercepting and exploiting them. Therefore, tele-nurses should strongly audit all of their current and available security measures and assess how to protect their patient privacy and protection through applying of policies. Most of tele-nurses are working for a hospital or organization which providing them by laptops with a recent and very high level of security and encryption, so that hackers and/or other outside sources cannot intercept patients' confidential sensitive and personal information [11].

Currently, the Health Insurance Portability and Accounting Act (HIPAA) summarize rules and regulations discussing how nurses and healthcare providers protect patients' personal data through storing and sharing. HIPAA declares that patients' identifiable information should to be encrypted so that only the nurses and other healthcare professionals involved in patients' care can access it. In addition to, many other considerations related to the patients' confidentiality and safety of their clinical data [10, 11].

5. Types of telenursing delivery models in nursing practice

Mainly, there are three types of Telenursing delivery models. The *first model* is storing and forwarding technologies to enable transferring of diagnostic imaging and physiologic data starting with digitally generated, stored then transferred as needed, without necessary of patient's presence. For example, vital signs, lab results, diagnostic tests such as MRI, CT, ultrasound and x-rays. *Second model* is live videoconferencing which is carried out by using of advanced telecommunication technologies such as virtual two-way, real-time using computers, microphones, audio and video transfer. It can be used for live visits specially for mental health, urgent care, patient education and other care management. Remote monitoring is the *third model*, using remotely for monitoring patients through digital technology to collect medial information then transmitting it to other specified healthcare providers at another location which named as Center for Connected Health Practice (CCHP). *Fourth model* is mobile health (MHealth) which means using of smart phones or mobile devices in healthcare provision. It means that any nursing care or health services can be provided through a combination of all or some of the other telehealth types. For example, using of mobile devices in patients' home which can transmit daily vitals, lab results for more frequent access to care, as diabetes and cardiac diseases [12].

6. Role of telenursing services in decreasing global nursing shortage

The shortage of healthcare team members all over the world can be decreased, especially among nurses through widely promoting the use of telenursing in providing so many services as the following:

- **Home care:** One of the most distinctive applications of telenursing is home care. The most intended target is elderly patients and others with special needs. For example, immobilized patients, or live in remote areas or difficult to reach services, citizens with chronic ailments, as chronic obstructive pulmonary disease (COPD), diabetes mellitus, congestive heart disease, or neural degenerative diseases as Parkinson's disease, Alzheimer's disease and ALS, its preferable to stay at home and be regularly visited and assisted by telenursing apps via videoconferencing, internet or videophone. Those apps enable nurses to receive real information about patients' status, coordinate care at home and ensure care management changes. In traditional home care, a nurse can visit up to five to seven clients per day. By using telenursing, a nurse can visit around 12–16 patients per day [13].

- **Telephone triage:** It refers to the clinically-based calls related to symptoms. Clinicians assess symptoms by asking the patient detailed questions about illness or injury. The main task of clinician is to estimate the urgent symptoms. They also use pattern recognition, as well as other problem-solving processes. Clinicians may utilize different guidelines, via paper or electronic formats to determine the urgency of symptoms. Telephone triage requirement is to evaluate symptoms and provide health guidance and advice which guides patients to advanced level of care (emergent, urgent, or non-urgent) according to their general condition and symptoms. Home self-care management can be provided through telephone triage staff; also medical advices can be provided for non-urgent patients at home. It may involve health education for patients. Telephone triage can be applied in settings as emergency rooms, large call centers, ambulance services, clinics, physician offices and student health centers [11].

The main benefit of telephone triage services is decreasing the amount of non-emergent visits to ER or emergency departments. According to the high patient volumes, the waiting areas of emergency department may become overcrowded, resulting in many patients leaving ER without being seen. Telephone triage staff use the electronic health records which generated by a health system encounters. This ability to access patients' health records can help triage staff in evaluating the patient efficiently because of the provided information as allergies and comorbidities. Accessibility to patients' health records helps in providing demographic information which can allow the triage staff to send necessary emergency services for the patient. So that, telephone triage service can help in decreasing lower-acuity patient visits to ER an emergency department [14].

- **Case management:** A common application of telenursing and can be used by call centers and operated by managed care organizations, which are staffed by well-trained registered nurses who act the role of case managers or perform patient triage and counseling as an important mean of regulating patient's access [15].

- **Chronic disease management:** A telenursing applications are widely beneficial through the patients with chronic illnesses. Those apps can enhance adherence to the nursing care plan, help managing symptoms and control health parameters of patients (e.g., checking and/or reading patient's blood pressure and/or blood glucose level) and allow nurses to alleviate symptoms through remote instructions [15].

- **Pregnancy and newborn monitoring and care:** Through video communication, nurses can provide mothers with professional advice and guidance about pregnancy, conduct preparation courses about childbirth, monitor women and newborns' vitals (entered by a patient or detected by smart medical devices) [16].

- **Pre-postoperative patient care:** Nurses can track patients' vital signs by connecting some medical devices then communicate with patients through video calls to prepare them pre-surgical by guidance them. Also nurses can follow up pre-operative instructions with patients. Nurses' e-visits after surgery can facilitate recovery and help in identify possible exacerbations by using photos and videos sent to them by a patient [17].

- **Mental health:** Telenursing applications have also been utilized by psychiatric nurses in mental health. Tele-psychiatry is useful at many settings or environments within limited access to care, including emergency rooms, rural areas, crisis zones and natural disasters and during wars. This technology can facilitate delivering of mental health care in areas without any mental health care resources by conducting scheduled video calls with psychiatric nurses. The benefits of these video calls are improving patients with mental disorders medication adherence, identifying additional symptoms, reducing anxiety and stress and promoting patients' coping mechanisms. Much of the time, tele-psychiatric care requires involving of live interacting between patient and care giver. It can be occurred through video conference or video calls. Tele-psychiatry has the ability to improve patient-centered and integrated care, allowing for the establishing of different mental health resources into the treatment plan of the patient [18].

Using of technology in mental health has a significant impact on crisis management and suicide prevention. In addition to direct health care, telenursing and tele-psychiatry, some organizations as Crisis Text Line have established text chatting system into crisis therapy and adopted a new line of resources to be available for people in mental health crises. This is mainly for therapy than in-person or over phone and can be utilized by teens and adolescent for their mental health [19].

7. Telenursing and nursing informatics

Nursing informatics, as a main branch of health informatics, has happened delineated by Judith Rae Graves and Sheila Corcoran as "a mixture of computer and information science, and nursing sciences created to assist in the administration and processing of data, news, and information to support the practice of acting as a nurse and the transfer of care." Telenursing is a potential use of fostering sciences concerned with information and essentially, tending sciences concerned with information has dressed as a fault-finding environment idea allure growth [13].

8. Benefits of telenursing

Telenursing can solve the widely trend problem of nursing shortage. It provides easy accessibility of nurses to patients. Nurses can focus on their patients' care and satisfaction without the traditional on-site appointments, so efficiency will be improved. Nurses should use their skills of listening, critical thinking and assessment, which they used to do in traditional settings for supporting their patients. Although in-body first-contact medical care has a difference of benefits, the benefits of telenursing are solid for clients, registered nurses, and nurse experts. Among allure many benefits, telenursing grant permission help meet growing shortages of nurses; to weaken distances and sustain travel occasion, and to hold sufferers from emergency room. A better scope of task delight has existed recorded between tele-nurses [20].

8.1 Remote service delivery

Telehealth science admits nurse practitioners (NPs) to give medical aids by way of the computer network and traveling schemes. NPs give services utilizing differing forms, to a degree calculating, detached monitoring schemes, natural designs, and transfer guests. Telenursing blends visual and audio entertainment transmitted via radio waves, video, and paragraph-located news. NPs have equal understand; that the value of telehealth aid parallels that of in-person commission visits. Telehealth finishes considerably increase adeptness for NPs the one transfer service to customers in country societies and simply inhabited extents. The same electronics admits NPs to steadily monitor victims' well-being environments. For this, NPs engage peripheral maneuvers that succeed usual healing instruments in the way that stethoscopes, thermometers, and ancestry pressure cuffs [12].

8.2 Financial savings

The health systems' industry benefits considerably from telenursing in many important approaches. It reduces costs by decreasing emergency visits and hospital admissions. It is also useful in managing the chronic illnesses and improving nurses' utilization throughout most of hospital departments. Telenursing can humble costs for two together sufferers and experts. A 2017 study from Health Affairs erect that, approximately, a commission visit cost cases $146 while the cost of telehealth visit is only $79. Savings still contain lowered visit expenses and output gains from dropped attendant absences. Telemedicine's overall worth proper to surpass $64.1 billion by 2025, in accordance with Global Market Insights [21].

8.3 Improved bed allocation

By reconstructing effect choose extreme-risk customers—to a degree never-ending ailment sufferers and recent surgical cases—healthcare providers have established that telenursing offers a form that reduces readmissions significantly. Some organizations have listened inmates in ship telehealth programs. They secondhand questionnaires and given fitness-connected instruction all week, making inquiries straightforwardly only accompanying those partners the one were further of the help all the while the ending [7].

8.4 Patient comfort

Three in four clients feel affluent accompanying telemedicine, accompanying comforting until the plan of telenursing continually. Clients exceptionally like the plan of freely achieve consultants that ability usually wait laboriously due accompanying additional cases. According to a study of Massachusetts General Hospital telehealth sufferers, written a piece American Journal of Managed Care, most sufferers sensed in essence fitness visits were more available than in-woman visits, in addition to 60% sensed in essence visits were no various in status from in-individual visits, and as well 80% would advise in essence visits to kin and companions. NPs use telehealth technology to determine customer comfort levels and react therefore. The electronics admits NPs to fix the individual touch that home doctor visits formerly supported. Care providers again use the science to give duties to cases' commissions, to subsidiary hospitals, or to some part that offers availability [22].

8.5 Increased opportunities of healthcare employment

Insurers revere telehealth cost stockpiles as a habit to give first-rate help at intensely shortened costs. Consumers inquire consultations to acquire news from care providers fast and prevent the nearly $100 billion in expenses produce by loss to comprehend care plans. Analysts forecast that experts will occurrence a sharp increase in the patient meetings they transfer done yearly over the next 5 years, someday transferring about 27 million yearlong consultations [23].

8.6 Remote areas accessibility by patients

Nearby 100 of rural hospitals ceased operations among 2010–2019, with various hundred more services through the country facing probability of closure, based on the declarations of National Rural Health Association. These closures are on account of society shifts and reserve misallocations. As physicians refrain location to country extents, and as patient conveyance management evolve more complex, questions accompanying care character and inclusion shortages are increasing. However, many trust that telenursing aids can go at a great distance in solving this crisis. Within telehealth services, hospitals of rural areas can reduce costs, expand coverage, and eliminate the waiting time spent till deliver services. Incidentally, this alike rationale applies to giving duties to cases in cultivating countries with its own government. Although customers can immediately sustain telemedicine take care of as little as $50, not all providers offer telehealth that authorizes cases to collect the cost stockpiles. With adequate support and functional unification though, inmates here and there can have the skill to approach telenursing aids free in the forthcoming future [24].

9. Telenursing in nursing education

The universal pandemic of COVID-19 obliged the world on widespread ratification of telehealth in tending practice and nursing e-learning. While healthcare providers altered their method of care from straight forwardly to e-learning in nursing education, tending programs used telehealth to accomplish practical hours. Before the universal COVID-19 pandemic, most nurses received telehealth preparation through their task, nurse residence, or companies entertaining the science. This approving the declaration of American Academy of Ambulatory Care Nursing (AAACN) in 2018, which reported that most nursing preparation occurs during their clinical orientation for different jobs or residency program, instead of their academic training. As a result, when the global society was in need to embrace telehealth and telenursing to face COVID-19 consequences, healthcare professionals, especially nurses, obliged to apply them without needed training [25].

Nurses erect themselves poorly trained for complying their arrangements of be fond of telehealth. Nursing programs can determine nursing students needs which mainly concentrated on the importance of more training to support the standard of care while guiding along route, over the noticed changes through the fruitful telenursing environment. So the educational nursing organizations have to mandate telenursing to be incorporated into all nursing curriculum [26].

Nursing education can adopt the telenursing training both in care providing and in nursing education which will be a worldwide trend in nursing science and can definitely help in decrease the gap of nursing shortage. Telenursing as a scientific practical method can provide a care or health services within some aspects which are completely unique and different. Telenursing not only practical method for providing nursing care, but also is an art in communication through applying of social etiquette in the management of patients' care including evaluation of them. Applying of legal considerations starting with the nursing license to perform tasks and duties, as well as confidentiality of patients' data to protect their privacy. The core of any care is comforting the patients, but in telenursing the core extended to the family members with a cultural competence through a social appreciating for the financial considerations as the health insurance coverage. Technology skills using mainly in telenursing and telehealth are including the ways to troubleshoot most issues of connectivity [27].

According to the American Nurses Association identifications for achieving effective telenursing program for providing a healthcare, its necessary to follow up four systematic phases. Those phases are starting with planning as a *first phase* for providing the service through telenursing then the *second phase* of preparing for it with checking of all facilities. Both first and second phases are involving setting up in addition to implementing the telenursing program. The *third phase* is providing the service using any of the suitable telenursing types, and finally performance evaluation as the *fourth phase* is important to evaluate the quality of care, communication and client satisfaction [28].

Telenursing educational programs are slightly different from telenursing using in providing a healthcare mainly. Telenursing educational programs focus on the first and fourth phases, providing and performance evaluation. The difference in providing phase is involving telenursing conduction through care coordination, triage, client education and monitoring. While, performance evaluation phase is assessing the factors that affect quality of telenursing program such as types of gathering data, tools for data collection and clients' feedback and outcome [29].

United Kingdom started the evolution of applying the telehealth and telenursing in both practical and educational fields with big support and collaboration of a multidisciplinary system. Starting with conducting of educational programs and carrying out of other specialized training programs for nurses and other health team members on the effective use of technology and software use with related operation, since even the actual use of Computerized Decision Support Systems (CDSS) in Europe. Those systems were helping in decision-making and facilitating standardized protocols that each patient is unique with varied situations. In UK, the first target users of this systems were general practitioners (GPs), then the practitioner nurses involved in the patients' advice lines through the nurse-led telephone service. These lines were implemented in different districts in UK and around as NHS Direct (NHSD) which applied in England, following by NHS Direct Wales (NHSDW) conducted in Wales as well as NHS 24 in Scotland. All of those programs were based mainly on well-designed educational programs for the nurses [30].

Telenursing and telehealth simulations and clinicians on different clinical settings are using three stages of preparing, telenursing visit and debriefing. The preparation stage in telehealth allows nursing students to search in patient conditions, reviews the key nursing skills and plan for their needs to address during the call. Students should confirm the patient consent, ask all available questions and record all data during the visit. The debriefing phase evaluates the process of assessment, patient's general condition, communication skills and outcomes of the telenursing or telehealth visit [25].

The paper of National Organization of Nurse Practitioner Faculty (NONPF) published in 2018, supporting telenursing in the educational programs of nurse practitioner (NP). They provided general guidelines of strategies, competencies, and evaluation process for telenursing modalities incorporation within the NP curriculum. This paper recommended by the need for telenursing competencies in nursing schools and teaching nursing students the clinical skills and technology [31].

10. Global using of telenursing during COVID 19 pandemic

Although telehealth and telenursing are not new concepts, their use became widely necessary and popular with the appearance of COVID-19 pandemic. So many societal changes are globally occurring science the rise of COVID-19 pandemic. All of these global changes lead the health field to create new ways for providing care with promoting of social distancing as possible, quarantining as needed and preservation of some limited hospital services [32].

Using of telehealth and telenursing as a response to cover the patients' needs during COVID-19 pandemic in not only inside the strong financial countries' healthcare systems, but also through the developed countries systems according to their available resources. In the United States, definitely on March 27, 2020, some legislations were passed in order to protect both patients and healthcare providers through the growth of telenursing capabilities in the country. Also the CDC reported that possibility of telehealth use is very recommended to eliminate the spread of COVID-19. Applying of telenursing enables the country from keeping the high-risk patients' safety in their homes and receiving their routine care at the same time. Telenursing also allows Corona Virus positive nurses with mild symptoms to continue caring patients online from home [33].

Telenursing has significantly raised during the COVID-19 pandemic, because it can increase the social distancing by eliminating the patients' need for traveling and going to crowded areas. Decreasing the cost of personal protective equipment (PPE) as vital needs for health team is another benefit of telenursing. The benefits of telenursing during this pandemic can promote infection control, connect health team from different regions and allow rapid triage [34].

Before the COVID 19 pandemic, a limited sector of the general workforce was working occasionally from home. In the European Union (EU), the incidence of home-based teleworking and the combined mobile telework especially in providing of healthcare services was varied around 30% in Denmark, Netherlands and Sweden and nearby 10% in Czech Republic, Greece, Italy and Poland [35]. According to important findings of a study, the United States workforce that are working distance from home or through another alternative location reached about 20%, 16% in Japan and just only 1.6% in Argentina [36].

Based on applying of the global social distancing strategies, almost 4 between 10 employees in Europe used teleworking. Also health team members starting to use telehealth and telenursing in order to face the shortage of workforce especially in nurses. Other ways of teleworking started to be appeared as mobile health and monitoring [37]. The most noticed increase in teleworking was in the most affected countries by Corona virus, and based on where well developed teleworking was before the pandemic as in Finland, Luxembourg, the Netherlands, Belgium, Denmark, Ireland, Italy, Austria and Sweden by 40–60%. Also telehealth and telenursing were applied in Japan using the most recent robotic system and very advanced artificial intelligence technological devices [34].

Using of telehealth and telenursing during COVID-19 pandemic also appeared through the Middle East and inside the Arab countries with their different healthcare systems according to their available resources. In Egypt, telehealth and telenursing were applied using new technological devices which affected positively on the health care system in decreasing the patients' waiting list, increasing the health team members' efficacy and limiting the work burden on them. It reflected on the number of patients' visits to different outpatient clinics which decreased to 50% specifically in family medicine clinics [38].

In Saudi Arabia, the Ministry of Health applied "Seha," the e-health application which is free of charge, to enhance the healthcare system. This App support the visual medical consultations and apply face to face medical consultations for all citizens with their doctors anywhere across KSA. The "Seha" application was providing audio-video communication any time even through the weekends. In United Arab Emirates, the health care delivery system established telematics and telemedicine applications among 50% of hospitals for the long term provision of healthcare services. Through those hospitals, 90% of doctors and nurses providing healthcare by using smartphones and medical applications. Several UAE companies already provide telehealth services through different applications such as Health at Hand, TruDoc 24×7 and InstaPract. Also health insurance companies discovered that telehealth services can reduce healthcare costs [38] .

Figure 1 clarifies the Data Bridge Market Research report and related expectation belonging the huge growing in telehealth market of Middle East and Africa from 2022 and forecast to 2029, by type as software, hardware, systems and telecommunication. This growing also will be appeared in delivery modes as cloud-based delivery mode, on premise delivery mode and web-based delivery mode. The market of applications on smart phones or other electronic devices also in continuing growing involving general consultation, Gynecology, Cardiology Pathology, radiology, dermatology and others. So the end user of all the previous types and examples of telehealth and telenursing technologies will be reflected on growing the international market of hospital telehealth, home telehealth & telenursing and/or physician telehealth [39].

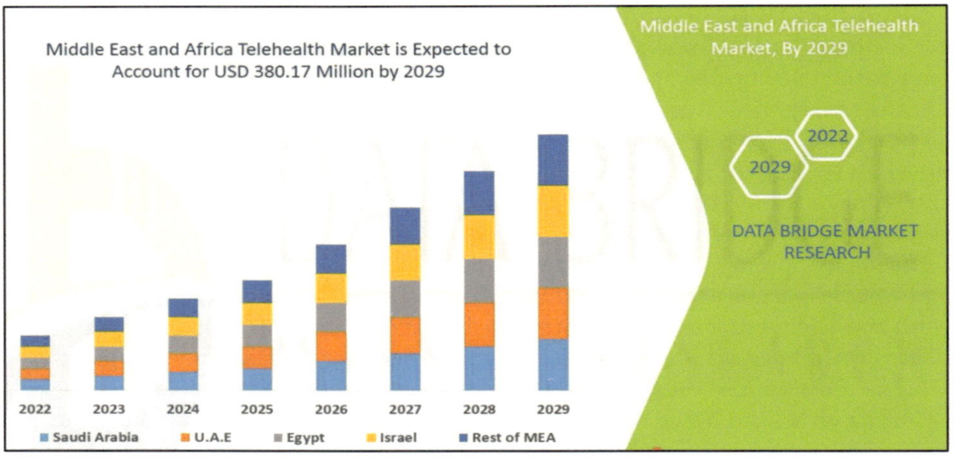

Figure 1.
Data Bridge, Market Research, Market Analysis Study: 2022. Published Report, Middle East and Africa Telehealth Market. https://www.databridgemarketresearch.com/reports/middle-east-and-africa-telehealth-market.

11. Telenursing development in worldwide nursing research

Up to date major nursing researches in telenursing are still focusing publication on the developed countries mainly as the United States, Canada and the United Kingdom which mainly still leading the field. The main findings of those major telenursing researches appear a positive significant association between the telenursing development's level and the technological development levels of countries. Different telenursing trials in such developed countries have proven that integrating of telenursing into the mainstream of their healthcare delivery systems is feasible and very beneficial [40].

There are so many telenursing trials all over the world which approved that mixed levels of efficacy could be reached among different age group of populations and through different healthcare dimensions as older adults' self-care management of many chronic illnesses, prenatal, natal and postnatal services specially in family planning counseling, surgical recovery, pediatric health care and emergency services. The majority of telenursing researches have demonstrated their outcomes of supporting the effectiveness of nursing care and related competencies, for reducing inaccessibility and contributing to nursing education, training and development [1].

Also nursing research based on telenursing trials in developing countries are presenting the same outcomes of those developed ones. As examples, applying of telenursing programs, trials and styles in nursing researches in such poor income African countries as Ghana, Nigeria, Ethiopia, Kenia, Egypt are detecting the big benefits and effectiveness of telenursing applications, mobile-based data, devices and other types in healthcare delivery system. Although the weak level of technological developments of developing countries, their findings were as the same line of other developed with nearly recommendations as many future researches in different telenursing dimensions as well as adding of telenursing education in the undergraduate and postgraduate curriculums [41].

Most recommendations of the recent telenursing research papers are focusing on the need for further research efforts be directed to theory-driven researches about communication, which will lead to effective telenursing process. Policy-makers and telenursing managers need to improve the management design of telenursing operations for optimizing of related efficacy and quality. Using of different telenursing models still in need to further research and developments to be adopted and integrated widely into the healthcare delivery system [19].

12. Advantages and disadvantages of telenursing

Telenursing concentrates on the communicating, organization and administration of care and/or duty resorting to information transfers novelty inside the field of fostering. Telenursing attendants take advantage of the nursing procedure to present prudence to individual patients or distinguished patient populaces over a telecom novelty. Imperatively, the nursing methodology and in consideration of practice are the unchanging in telenursing as in conventional nursing practice. Among the many miscellaneous clinical abilities of telenursing, nurses are observing subjects accompanying constant contaminations, share cases deal with their reactions and co-morbidities, and organizing administer to inmates the one require services from miscellaneous well-being experts [42]. Telenursing practitioners give nursing mind by:

- utilizing clinical formulas and calculations, conventions, or rules to evaluate the indications and patient needs efficiently;
- prioritizing the positive outcomes of patient needs;
- collaborating and establishing an arrangement of nursing care with patient and strong instructions, which may integrate different proposals for deliberation, back to directions and training; and
- assessing the overall conclusions.

- **Telenursing offers comfort:** Penciling in a midday meal-moment visit accompanying the doctor can explain experiment, specifically when a cannot-miss phone call assimilates the adulthood of your dim. Telemedicine simplifies this issue. Through feature, Web talk, or contact, professionals can entrance on a remedy or doom accompanying a doctor they have happened observing for completely a very long time if that doctor inexorably gives telenursing aids or accompanying another authority in their scheme. When a patient enrolls, he or she can contemplate out another in-order doctor's happening. The objective of telenursing searches out create an encounter that almost indicates an established technician visit [43].
- **Telenursing is cost-efficiency:** An extending number of professionals are taxing less for a telemedicine counsel than they would for an in-individual visit. Telemedicine can also decrease travel costs. This is specifically right for those filling a place limited groups. Provincial kins the one would always travel hours at a distance their approach to disturb key well-being duties attainable it from the solace of their comfortable armchair [21].
- **Telenursing advances safety in healthcare system:** Patients are certainly freed from the hospital more rapidly than at any additional be present at current memory before; accompanying differing cures and repeatedly failing to offer the learning they should nurture their condition convincingly. Telenursing permits these subjects to return home, which spares cash, nevertheless permits ruling

class expected supported by an expert until they are well or are handling their condition absolutely. Postoperative sufferers misuse backing, as they repeatedly have asking concerning what may be "common" that can certainly surrender care of by healing attendants, the one can resolve if a patient is attacking a complexity or a conventional effect of their resection. Telenursing gives a freedom net to patients the one can be struggling with handling their condition at home, averting complications that take care of because success being hospitalized again [44].

- **Telenursing guarantees less come into sight the robbing range:** Most crowd have thrown through that old age-old issue of us or People while property our mares to visualize our essential care doctor or dental professional. Telemedicine disposes concerning these methods. Online care is truly a massive part from our parts. It takes any minutes to record and set the well-being experiences in, and following you are qualified to take the government provision you demand, she suggests [45].

12.1 Disadvantages of telenursing

One of the important hindrances of appropriating telenursing from patient's viewpoint is patient secrecy. Persistent solitude and the freedom of private dossier must be protected, repaying little heed to the gathering plan used to collect dossier. Security and freedom is a superior thought in telenursing, and inmates and specialists must two together feel protected that dossier is gathered and kill fixedly [37].

- **Telenursing faces photoelectric errors:** Engineering is while hard as the electrical current that keeps it running. Severe trend and various disturbances can influence a force collapse or upset a netting partnership, muddling online argument accompanying a guru. Workers should get that above preparation online visits [43].

- **Telenursing faces the issue of incompetent amount:** While being intelligent to connect accompanying your essential foresight doctor or dental professional is a physical additionally, sure non-spoken prompts grant permission now sneak past the cracks. According to, skilled are no limits on in what way or manner you can utilize telenursing, unmistakably individual of the cons is you cannot mainly touch or feel the patient [46].

- **The adulthood of the more experienced cases has an issue accompanying integrity concerning this new design:** Telenursing maybe a hard pill to consume for more experienced subjects the one have existed not prepared machines and change as a companion to news and practice. As opposite to impression that they are, certainly "replaced" by machines, these experts should be influenced to view telenursing and telecom as a subordinate to expert practice. Studies have showed that most cases are intensely indulging of telenursing, still any specialists have existed more gradual to grasp this novelty. Nevertheless, telenursing is in this place to stay and will just cultivate, and experts the one grasp new architecture will find that their heap is brightened, and their subjects are more athletic and more completed by their care [47].

- **Telenursing faces the issue of material opposition:** The adulthood of fighting creates from doctors trying to assenting exploit the new engineering, still this disinclination just expands essentially. In the meantime, their interest has existed decided when they consider on the various habits they can start to use these electronics to survive the inmates the one have chronic deceases [42].

13. Barriers to telenursing practice

The adulthood of the more experienced subjects has an issue with integrity concerning this new construction: Telenursing maybe a hard dose to consume for more seasoned patients the one have happened not prepared machines and change as a companion to information and practice. As opposite to impression that they are, certainly "displaced" by machines, these masters should be swayed to view telenursing and telecom as. Current telenursing barriers can be summarized into the following [45]:

- Technology—restricted speedy broadband computer network.
- Cost—more prohibitive in detached districts.
- Licensure allowable limits on practice districts.
- Living with multiple never-ending environments.
- Those the one have less approach to connected to the internet money, from culturally and linguistically various backdrops.
- Reimbursement—depressed or lack of telehealth in few detached regions due to lack of compensation.
- Resistance—lack of buy-in; opposition to change, lack of count on electronics, lack of patient agreement and abilities.
- Provider skill sets, abilities deficient.
- Human calculating connect/utility—lack of calculating/telehealth literacy for example, sensitive patient groups.
- Olders, live rurally, have less precise education.
- Lower socioeconomic rank.

Despite the nurses' concerns about the results of bettering in telehealth and the potential affect nursing parts, the trustworthy and responsive science aided to overcome the barriers to agreement. Through telenursing, nurses supply distance feeding care, by listening, instruction, follow-up, detached dossier accumulation and attacks, pain administration, family support, and combining several branches of learning care in a creative habit [48].

14. Core competencies through telenursing skills

The main competencies, individual or more center competencies necessary for telenursing in major categories of [49]:

- coaching and ideas abilities,
- ability to connect clinical information,
- moral awareness,
- auxiliary attitude,
- comprehensive abilities such as examining, and
- implementation abilities.

Acknowledgements

Grateful thanks for Dr. Ahmed Abdel Hakim, Prof. Dr. Amira Elbeih and Prof. Dr. Hoda Zaki for their effective psychological and scientific support.

Conflict of interest

The authors declare no conflict of interest.

Author details

Zainab Attia Abdallah[1*], Engy Abdel Rahman Khamis[2], Fatma M. Ibrahim[3] and Ayiat Allah Wagdy Farag[1]

1 Community Health Nursing, Modern University for Technology and Information (MTI), Egypt

2 Medical Surgical Nursing, Modern University for Technology and Information (MTI), Egypt

3 RAK, Medical and Health Science University, Ras al Khaimah, United Arab Emirates

*Address all correspondence to: z.attia30@gmail.com

References

[1] Asimakopoulou E. Telenursing in clinical practice and education. International Journal of Caring Sciences. 2020;**13**(2):781-782

[2] Keshavaraz N, Naderifar M, Firouzkohi M, Abdollahimohammad A, Akbarizadeh MR. Effect of telenursing on the self-efficacy of patients with myocardial infarction: A quasi-experimental study. Signa Vitae. 2020;**16**(2):92-96

[3] Schaumberg L. Advanced practice telenursing through a pandemic. Journal of Psychosocial Nursing and Mental Health Services. 2020;**58**(9):4-6. DOI: 10.3928/02793695-20200624-09

[4] Galiero R, Pafundi PC, Nevola R, Rinaldi L, Acierno C, Caturano A, et al. The importance of telemedicine during COVID 19 pandemic: A focus on diabetic retinopathy. Journal of Diabetes Research. 2020:1-8. DOI: 10.1155/2020/9036847

[5] Dorsey ER, Topol EJ. Telemedicine 2020 and the next decade. The Lancet. 2020;**395**(10227):859

[6] Frey MB, et al. Considerations when using telemedicine as the advanced practice registered nurse. 2021. Available from: https://www.ncbi.nlm.nih.gov/pmc/articles/PMC7835535/

[7] Purabdollah M, Ghasempour M. Tele-nursing new opportunity for nursing care in covid-19 pandemic crisis. Iranian Journal of Public Health. 2020;**49**(1):130-131. DOI: 10.18502/ijph.v49iS1.3685

[8] Heo H, Lee K, Jung E, Lee H. Developing the first telenursing service for COVID-19 patients: The experience of South Korea. International Journal of Environmental Research and Public Health. 2021;**18**(13):6885. DOI: 10.3390/ijerph18136885

[9] Arneson SL, Tucker SJ, Mercier M, Singh J. Answering the call: Impact of tele-ICU nurses during the COVID-19 pandemic. Critical Care Nurse. 2020;**40**(4):25-31. DOI: 10.4037/ccn2020126

[10] Rutledge C, et al. Preparing nurses for roles in telehealth: Now is the time! 2021. Available from: https://ojin.nursingworld.org/MainMenuCategories/ANAMarketplace/ANAPeriodicals/OJIN/TableofContents/Vol-26-2021/No1-Jan-2021/Preparing-Nurses-for-Roles-in-Telehealth-Now-is-the-Time.html#Mataxen

[11] Jácome M, Rego N, Veiga P. Potential of a nurse telephone triage line to direct elderly to appropriate health care settings. Journal of Nursing Management. 2019;*27*(6):1275-1284. DOI: 10.1111/jonm.12809

[12] Muller AE, Berg RC, Jardim PS, Johansen TB, Ormstad SS. Can remote patient monitoring be the new standard in primary care of chronic diseases, post-COVID-19? Telemedicine and E-Health. 2021;**22**(1):453

[13] Ye J. The role of health technology and informatics in a global public health emergency: Practices and implications from the COVID-19 pandemic. JMIR Medical Informatics. 2020;**8**(7):e19866. DOI: 10.2196/19866

[14] Zhang N. How Coronavirus Accelerated the Rise of Telemedicine. CNBC; 2020

[15] Agastiya MC, Kurianto E, Akalili H, Wicaksana AL. The impact of telehealth on self-management of patients with type 2 diabetes: A systematic review on interventional studies. Diabetes & Metabolic Syndrome: Clinical Research & Reviews. 2022;**16**(5):102485

[16] Şat SÖ, Sözbir ŞY. Use of mobile applications by pregnant women and levels of pregnancy distress during the COVID-19 (coronavirus) pandemic. Maternal and Child Health Journal. 2021;**25**(7):1057-1068. DOI: 10.1007/s10995-021-03162-y

[17] Sato D. Effectiveness of telenursing for postoperative complications in patients with prostate cancer. Asia-Pacific Journal of Oncology Nursing. 2020;**7**(4):396-403. DOI: 10.4103/apjon.apjon_28_20

[18] Zhou X, Snoswell CL, Harding LE, Bambling M, Edirippulige S, Bai X, et al. The role of telehealth in reducing the mental health burden from COVID-19. Telemedicine Journal and E-Health. 2020;**26**(4):377-379. DOI: 10.1089/tmj.2020.0068

[19] Chakeri A, Jalali E, Ghadi MR, Mohamadi M. Evaluating the effect of nurse-led telephone follow-ups (tele-nursing) on the anxiety levels in people with coronavirus. Journal of Family Medicine and Primary Care. 2020;**9**(10):5351-5354. DOI: 10.4103/jfmpc.jfmpc_847_20

[20] Fronczek AE, Rouhana NA. Attaining mutual goals in telehealth encounters: Utilizing King's framework for telenursing practice. Nursing Science Quarterly. 2018;**31**(3):233-236. DOI: 10.1177/0894318418774884

[21] Eurofound. COVID-19 Could Permanently Change Teleworking in Europe. Dublin: Eurofound; 2020

[22] Sakinah S, Nurdin S. Telenursing and self-management among patient with hypertension. Malahayati International Journal of Nursing and Health Science. 2021;**3**(2):103-109

[23] Euro found and ILO. Working Anytime, Anywhere: The Effects on the World of Work. Luxembourg and Geneva: Publications Office of the European Union and ILO; 2017

[24] Herliani YK, Shabrina AP, Andrini NP, Melawardani AF, Rahmi HA, Maulana MR. The effectiveness of telenursing on the patient's quality of life: A review. Jurnal Ilmu Keperawatan: Journal of Nursing Science. 2021;**9**(2):212-218. DOI: 10.21776/ub.jik.2021.009.02.9

[25] American Academy of Ambulatory Care Nursing (AAACN). Scope and Standards of Practice for Professional Telehealth Nursing. 6th ed. Anthony J. Jannetti, Inc; 2018

[26] American Association of Colleges of Nursing (AACN). AACN Essentials. AACN Education Resources. Washington: The Voice of Academic Nursing; 2020. Available from: https://www. aacnnursing.org/Education-Resources/ AACN-Essentials

[27] Hargreaves L, et al. COVID-19 pandemic impact on nursing student education: Telenursing with virtual clinical experiences. 2021. Available from: https://www.ncbi.nlm.nih.gov/pmc/articles/PMC8529906/

[28] Guenther J, et al. Five steps to integrating telehealth into APRN curricula. 2021. Available from:https://www.sciencedirect.com/science/article/pii/S1555415520306462

[29] Digin F, Zeynep KO. Telehealth and telenursing in COVID-19 pandemic. Turkiye Klinikleri Journal of Nursing

Sciences. 2021;**13**(4). DOI: 10.5336/nurses.2020-80858

[30] Elliott AM, McAteer A, Heaney D, Ritchie LD, Hannaford PC. Examining the role of Scotland's telephone advice service (NHS 24) for managing health in the community: Analysis of routinely collected NHS 24 data. BMJ Open. 2015

[31] Hilty DM, Maheu MM, Drude KP, Hertlein KM. The need to implement and evaluate telehealth competency: Frameworks to ensure quality care across behavioral health professions. Academic Psychiatry. 2018;**42**(6):818-824. DOI: 10.1007/s40596-018-0992-5

[32] Piscesiana E, Afriyani T. The effect of tele-nursing on preventing re-admission among patients with heart failure: A literature review. International Journal of Nursing and Health Services. 2020;**3**(2):251-260

[33] CDC. Coronavirus Disease 2019 (COVID-19). USA: Centers for Disease Control and Prevention; 2020

[34] Dooley B. Japan needs to telework. Its paper-pushing offices make that hard. The New York Times. 2020

[35] ILO. Keys for Effective Teleworking During the COVID 19 Pandemic. Geneva: International Labour Office; 2020

[36] ILO. In the Face of a Pandemic: Ensuring Safety and Health at Work. Geneva: International Labour Office; 2020

[37] WHO. WHO Announces COVID-19 Outbreak a Pandemic. 2020.Available from: http://www.euro.who.int/en/health-topics/health-emergencies/coronavirus-covid 19/news/news/2020/3/who announces-covid-19-outbreak-a-pandemic

[38] Middle East and Africa Telehealth Market. Industry Trends and Forecast to 2029. Published Report, Data Bridge, Market Research. 2022

[39] Wong AK, Bayuo J, Wong FK, Yuen WS, Lee AY, Chang PK, et al. Effects of a nurse-led telehealth self-care promotion program on the quality of life of community-dwelling older adults: Systematic review and meta-analysis. Journal of Medical Internet Research. 2022;**24**(3):e31912

[40] Imenokhoeva M. Telehealth in the European Union: Improving Access to Healthcare. Patient Access, Emerging Technologies, Care, Technology; 2020

[41] Ellatif AE-SA, Elsayed DMS, Abosree TH. Knowledge and attitude of faculty of nursing students regarding telenursing. Journal of Nursing Science. 2023;**4**(1):677-689

[42] Wright CH, Wright J, Shammassian B. COVID-19: Launching neurosurgery into the era of telehealth in the United States. World Neurosurgery. 2020;**140**:54-55. DOI: 10.1016/j.wneu.2020.05.092

[43] El Jamal N, Abi-Saleh B, Isma'eel H. Advances in telemedicine for the management of the elderly cardiac patient. Journal of Geriatric Cardiology. 2021;**18**(9):759-767

[44] Wijesooriya NR, Mishra V, Brand PLP, Rubin BK. COVID-19 and telehealth, education, and research adaptations. Paediatric Respiratory Reviews. 2020;**35**:38-42. DOI: 10.1016/j.prrv.2020.06.009

[45] Rezaie F, Firouzkouhi M, Abdollahimohammad A, Naderifar M. Comparing the effect of education through SMS with face-to-face method on awareness and care in mothers with premature neonates. Medical Science. 2019;**23**(98):540-546

[46] Razu SR, Yasmin T, Arif TB, Islam MS, Islam SM, Gesesew HA, et al. Challenges faced by healthcare professionals during the COVID-19 pandemic: A qualitative inquiry from Bangladesh. Frontiers in Public Health. 2021;**9**:647315

[47] Firouzkouhi M, Abdollahimohammad A, Arulappan J, Nouraei T, Farzi J. Challenges and opportunities of using telenursing during COVID-19 pandemic: An integrative review. Frontiers in Health Informatics. 2021;**10**(1):98. DOI: 10.30699/fhi.v10i1.332

[48] Bashir A, Bastola DR. Perspectives of nurses toward telehealth efficacy and quality of health care: Pilot study. JMIR Medical Informatics. 2018;**6**(2):e35

[49] Caetano R, Silva AB, Guedes AC, Paiva CC, Ribeiro GD, Santos DL, et al. Challenges and opportunities for telehealth during the COVID-19 pandemic: Ideas on spaces and initiatives in the Brazilian context. Cad Saúde Pública. 2020;**36**:e00088920. DOI: 10.1590/0102-311X00088920

Section 2

Teaching and Learning

Chapter 4

Embedding the Humanities into Nursing Education

Mei-Yu Yeh

Abstract

Humanistic education in nursing began in the 1980s. At that time, nursing education emphasized the human being and regarded each person as a unique individual with potential. However, modern developments in medical technologies and changes in the health-care environment have led to a trend toward dehumanization of the healthcare industry. Various developments, particularly in genetics, have raised issues related to human dignity, value, and ethics. The development of a humanized care model based on both scientific principles and a humanistic ideal has become an urgent issue in today's professional nursing education environment. A humanistic education in the nursing profession will allow nurses to develop a broader perspective, to cultivate insight, to understand and to feel the unique experience of patients, and to look at problems from multiple perspectives, especially in complex situations. The challenge of today's nursing education is using multiple teaching strategies to improve humanistic cultivation of humanities education in the nursing profession.

Keywords: cultivation, humanities, humanistic education, nursing, nursing education

1. Introduction

In addition to the COVID-19 pandemic severely affecting healthcare services worldwide, the innovation of high-tech and precision medical resources in the twenty-first century has also greatly improved. This improvement and innovation will also change the future medical care environment and trends [1]. Moreover, the nursing profession in this new era of information and biotechnology development has been affected by technological developments and is bound to continue to be affected by ever-changing scientific and technological achievements, of which genetics raises issues related to human dignity, values, and ethics [2]. Rapid changes in medical technologies have resulted in dehumanization of the healthcare industry [2]. Although compassion is a core value of the nursing profession, the decline of compassion in the broader medical environment has led to a similar decline in this core value in the nursing profession. The nursing profession will face unprecedented challenges if nurses cannot embody empathy and compassion when caring for patients [3]. How to develop and provide a humanized care model based on science and humanities has become an urgent issue in today's professional nursing education [4–6].

The value of humanistic education to the nursing profession is to provide an affective experience of humanity, care, and esthetic appreciation; to develop broader perspectives; to cultivate insight; to help nurses understand and feel the unique experience of patients; and to look at problems from multiple perspectives, especially in complex life situations. The challenge of today's nursing education is how to use multiple teaching strategies to improve humanistic cultivation in the nursing profession's humanities education. However, modern nursing education focuses on acquiring professional knowledge and ignores cultivating a humanist spirit. In order to help nurses, adapt to the rapidly changing medical environment and express professional and humanistic caring, the six Es framework (Example, Explanation, Exhortation, Environment, Experience, and Expectation) should be promoted in humanistic-nursing education [3, 6].

2. The meaning of "Humane" or the "Humanities"

In Confucian thought, the term "humane" connotes benevolence, righteousness, morality, and etiquette. These characteristics regulate the relationships between "people and themselves," "people and others," "people and society," "people and nature," and "people and the supernatural." Compared with the East's Confucian humanistic thinking, the West was very eager to get rid of the bondage of God during the Renaissance, develop humanism, and establish thinking with "people" as the central concept. At that time, it followed the example of ancient Greece and Rome, focusing on the Seven Liberal Arts (grammar, rhetoric, dialectic, arithmetic, geometry, astronomy, and music), and advocating liberal education [7].

From the perspective of historical development, this can be called "humanistic education." After the Renaissance and the Reformation, the core value of humanism, with people at the core, remained unchanged. Comparing the aforementioned connotations of the "humanities" and "humaneness' in the East and the West, humanistic thought in the East is influenced by mainstream Confucianism, emphasizing the "interpersonal norms of benevolence, righteousness, morality, etiquette, and ethics." By contrast, Western humanities take "people as the main body of thinking" and centers on people as the thing to be valued. In short, humanity includes three aspects. The first aspect refers to human thinking, which involves respecting oneself and the value of human life. The second aspect refers to the viewpoint of inter-subjectivity between human beings, emphasizing that people should respect each other. The third aspect refers to the establishment of a harmonious relationship between people and society [7].

Humanitas in Latin means humanity and upbringing. Humanistic care is the exercise of the humanistic spirit and having a humanistic spirit is having the ability to become attached to others and to have the courage to love and care for people. It includes the ability to be inspired to change thoughts or behaviors and to connect with others and make them feel the power and mystery of life [8]. Humanistic literacy regulates relationships between people of various ethnic groups, cultures, genders, and beliefs. Humanistic literacy can make up for aspects that science cannot cover, including encouraging critical reflection on technology, preventing overspecialization, and arresting tendencies toward dehumanization. Humanities and social sciences can include literature, art, philosophy, history, sociology, ethics, etc. Literature and the arts provide opportunities for individuals to describe their feelings and observations to understand suffering, the situations of others, and the essence of human nature. It can also heighten insight into other people's responsibilities and improve the core competencies of caring, such as observation and analysis, empathy, self-awareness, and reflection [9, 10]. Throughout history, nurses have established their profession's position and role in society and confirmed the value of their contributions. Sociology helps to understand the nursing profession's place in a cultural and social context and the effect of culture on healthcare behaviors [11]. Ethical inquiry helps nurses cultivate their moral sensitivities and become practitioners of reasonable care [12]. When the humanities and social sciences are integrated into professional teaching, the improvement of humanistic literacy will naturally give rise to a uniformity in the actions of nursing staff and realize the purpose of humanistic education [13].

3. Importance of humanities education in nursing

Humanities are one of nursing's professional competencies. Nurses must have a human touch to ensure the physical and mental well-being of patients. In the process of patient care, nurses must have humanistic literacy to see the human side of the patient; reflecting and implementing humane care are the basis for the physical and mental healing of patients and is one of the nursing profession's core values. Therefore, a lack of compassion in nursing education may lead to clinical care being dominated by a conception of patients as mere objects to be subjected to medical instruments and procedures without any voice of their own [3]. Therefore, nursing staff must develop the ability to be aware of the unique experiences of patients [14]. In addition to teaching professional knowledge, nursing education should cultivate compassion to assist nurses to be empathetic [15, 16]. When nurses face the humanistic needs of care recipients, they use their emotional awareness and reflection to develop a sense of themselves and their patients' life stories. It is necessary to activate the energy of humanistic nursing care through systematic teaching strategies [17, 18] to enhance nurses' cultivation of humanism in their own lives and express the humanistic spirit of caring, concern, and compassion in nursing [8, 19].

Calman pointed out that allowing nursing students to experience other people's life experiences can increase their own sensitivity to others' suffering [20–23]. Reflecting on their own and their patients' life stories can help nurses to be more compassionate. Through empathy and reflection, nursing students can enhance their understanding of patients' life experiences, promote empathy, and improve their literacy to face complex situations [9, 10, 24–26]. Then, nursing students can internalize the characteristics of humanistic care. William Osler, the father of American medicine, believed that a good doctor must possess the humanistic qualities of the 3Hs: humility, humanity, and humor. These three humanistic qualities align with society's expectations for humanistic medical care [27]. Humanistic care is a core value of the nursing profession. A qualified nurse must be able to empathize with patients and understand their unique life experiences. Only a compassionate nurse can care for patients and provide humane care [28]. The nurses that impress patients the most are those who are respectful, empathetic, caring, professional, sensitive, and enthusiastic [3].

Through qualitative in-depth interviews, Yeh found that for the nursing profession, the essence of nursing humanities includes caring, respect, enthusiasm, and professional sensitivity. Among these, "caring" is the most important humanistic-nursing characteristic, which refers to having "empathy" or "sympathy" and being able to "show compassion from the heart." In addition to caring, respect is essential in the nursing profession because respect is the process of interaction; respect can correct an indifferent attitude and show self-discipline and politeness. Furthermore, a qualified nurse must possess professionalism sensitivity. In addition to having professional knowledge and skills, nurses also need to observe keenly, synchronize with patients, be emotionally present, understand, and interpret the patient's body language and nonverbal meanings, and help solve the patient's problems in a timely manner. At that point, the beauty of nursing humanities will also be fully displayed [29].

The development of the nursing profession should focus on humanistic education and be committed to caring for the whole human being. Nursing professionals must empathize with patients to help them. Understanding a sick "person" goes beyond reading instruments and performing routines; it involves perceiving a truly complete and living "person" with pain, expectations, and anxieties. In addition to the scientific and objective understanding of "disease," the understanding of "human beings" must rely on subjective life experience and feelings, putting oneself in the shoes of others, empathizing with them, and treating patients professionally and confidently with humanity and wisdom. Therefore, the meaning and substance of humanities are emphasizing human dignity and value, and the "human being" is the main body of scientific knowledge [3].

4. Teaching strategies in humanities education

The nursing profession needs to strengthen the knowledge and depth of humanities education. To encourage compassion among nursing staff, Ryan's 6Es (Example, Explanation, Exhortation, Environment, Experience, Expectation) should be used as the framework [30] for education in school and work environments to deepen the humanistic essence of nursing education (**Figure 1**). The 6Es include role modeling (Example), inspiration (Explanation), exhortation, and encouragement (Exhortation), the shaping of the environment (Environment), reflection on experiences (Experience), and self-expectation (Expectation). Since the deepening of

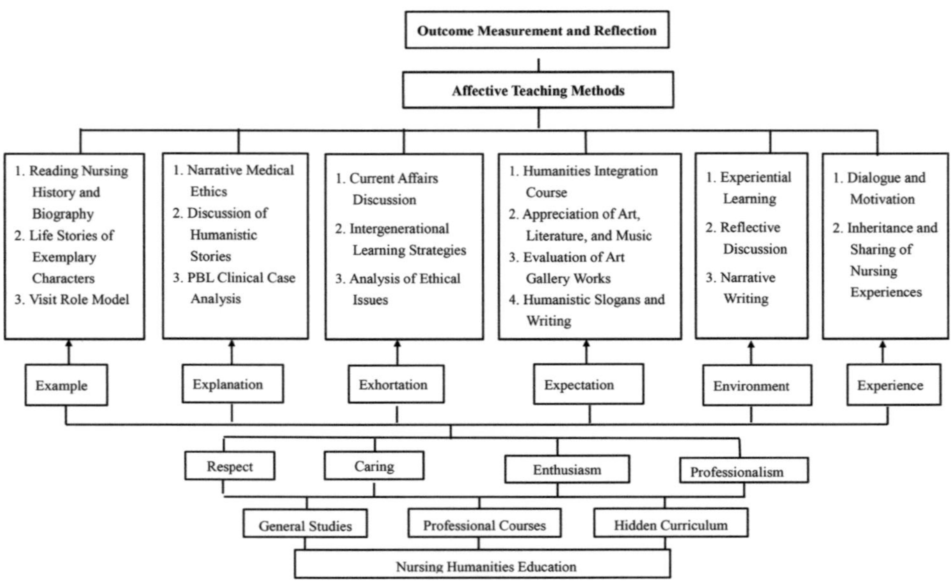

Figure 1.
Framework of humanistic-nursing education.

humanistic cultivation focuses on affective education, the use of 6Es in the cultivation of nursing humanistic essence aims to emphasize the recognition of intrinsic value, which internalizes the essence of human nature to the characteristics of nurses, and then engages the humanistic spirit [3, 6]. The 6Es involve the following: (1) Example: The humanistic connotation of nursing education must subtly implement humanistic care into nursing practice. Therefore, it is encouraged to use real figures in life as learning models so students can learn from example, (2) Explanation: Education should not be dogmatic or only require rote memorization. Instead, educators should encourage dialog, discussions of values, and reflection on why the nursing profession should be compassionate, what the core values are, and how nurses can implement and practice compassionate behaviors, (3) Exhortation: A compassionate spirit should be practiced through a variety of activities, such as video, story, and experience, (4) Environment: Compassionate and ethical values should be promoted on campus, (5) Experience: Experiential-learning activities should be arranged for nurses to practice providing compassionate care, and (6) Expectation: Nurses should be encouraged to set humanistic care goals to motivate themselves and continually pursue growth [3, 6].

Derbyshire pointed out that, in addition to using the 6Es teaching strategy, we can improve the inner awareness of nursing staff and discover our shared humanity through reading literary works, such as biographies, novels, and works on history and philosophy [31]. Literary descriptions of human life experiences can help caregivers feel and appreciate other people's life stories, including experiences involving illness, pain, anxiety, and the loss of function. When cultivated in literature and art, nursing staff can enrich their values through inner imagination, esthetic appreciation, and experience with care. In particular, the affective experience at the perceptual level can help nurses better implement the ideals of humanistic care [32]. Through the experience of reading literature and the observation of art, nursing staff can improve their observational skills; through the appreciation of music and drama, nurses can express their thoughts and feelings; through values clarification, identification of ethical values, and moral reflection, nurses can enhance their understanding of patients' life experience and enrich the nursing curriculum. Through narrative medicine, by listening to the life stories described by patients, nurses can understand diseases from the perspectives of patients [33–35]. Self-awareness and reflection stimulate nursing staffs' empathy, motivates them to learn, cultivates humanistic qualities, and brings humanity back to medical education [5, 9, 10, 36].

This study identified that intergenerational narrative inquiry can effectively improve the quality of humanistic care in nursing students [37]. Nursing students can change patients' perspectives on chronic diseases by understanding life stories of the elderly, inspiring students with a humanistic attitude, and deepening students' self-awareness. Through empathetic understanding, communication between generations can improve, which generate more positive attitudes toward the elderly from the students [37]. It helps nursing students to understand patients and illuminate the intricacy of specific phenomena and the paradigms that shape peoples' experiences [38]. Therefore, the storytelling process is a fundamental element of the narrative approach, as it provides the opportunity for reflective dialog [39], which allows for the acquisition and transfer of tacit knowledge [40, 41]. Each generation has different beliefs and memories, affected by different social background factors, and a generation gap is unavoidable [42], especially for younger nursing professionals [43–45]. Therefore, it is necessary to promote awareness and insight for different generations of nursing students, to enable the students to integrate previous learning and life experience, stimulate learning motivation, and establish intergenerational relationships. Through understanding patients' perspectives, nursing professionals learn to respect the emotional experience and exercise the empathetic side of human nature when caring for patients suffering from disease [16, 46].

5. Teaching plan design of nursing humanities

In order to deepen the humanistic care of nursing students, nursing education should be dedicated to improving humanistic qualities, helping nursing students to develop the ability to understand and feel the unique experience of patients, so that they can provide "patient-centered" humanized care in medical situations with humanistic caring skills. Especially in clinical practice, when facing the needs of patients, nursing staff must perceive and reflect on their own emotions through teaching, and develop a vision of seeing themselves and seeing the suffering of patients, which is the driving force behind professional care. In order to inspire students to have such reflections, we take students as the focus and discuss issues such as how to develop humanistic qualities of nursing students. Through group discussion and independent learning activities, students place their subjectivity in classrooms and clinical fields, think about the knowledge of nursing and humanities, and then enlighten the practice of humanistic actions. This is a student-centered perspective on humanistic cultivation and the design and practice of nursing humanistic teaching programs, which can better meet the needs of nursing education and clinical practice.

5.1 The design process of the nursing humanities teaching program

Since the humanistic spirit emphasizes the ability of empathy, it must be based on one's own life experience and generate a common understanding between people. Therefore, the design concept of the nursing humanities teaching program is to explore the students' self-growth experience and regional environment as the starting point for the cultivation of nursing humanities. Therefore, the design of the "Nursing Humanities" teaching program starts with students as the main body. First, let students talk about their own experiences, understand the inner structure of people, and stack up their unique inner spirit and world meaning. Finally, the students reflect on their own humanistic nursing care. Each nursing student brings their own life growth memory and integrates the humanistic elements in this course, initiating and shaping the students' outline to become modern humanistic care nurses.

The design process of the nursing humanities teaching program [29] includes the following: (1) Recruit 19 students who voluntarily participate in the group. Through group discussion dialog, reflection on homework, learning experience, and teacher participation in action and reflection, we constructed the core concepts and connotations of the nursing humanities teaching program. It includes three core concepts: life resilience generated through connections between people and the land, recognizing people's spiritual value from narration and stories, and modern nursing role models, (2) Constructing evaluation tools for nursing humanistic teaching programs, including the assessment of nursing humanistic practice, thematic study sheet, clinical practice experience narrative and reflection form, and peer quality assessment, as the evaluation tools of this teaching program, (3) In the fourth grade of the university's nursing department, the elective course "Nursing Humanities" is offered. There are three classes in total, with 61, 32, and 60 students taking the courses. Among them,

32 elective students are nursing students with clinical work experience, and (4) In the course of nursing humanities, through the narration of the nursing students' life experience, humanistic activity experience, and the process of critical reflection, with teaching strategies such as group discussion, dialog, and self-reflection, it can increase the breadth and depth of humanistic care, help nursing students have the ability to understand and feel the unique experience of patients, and provide students with clues to reflect on their future nursing careers.

5.2 Nursing humanities teaching program

The framework of the nursing humanities teaching program [3] is based on the life experience of nursing students themselves as the starting point of humanistic inspiration; second, they discuss the meaning of nursing humanities and the analysis of clinical nursing images. Then through the narration of the story, added humanistic elements, including the nourishment of humanistic images to explore the media material of the life value story (The Memory Keeper's Daughter), let students reflect on and experience the value of being human again. It is not only about a biological science viewpoint but also a rich humanistic and social context. Guided by the media mentioned above, nursing students can imagine people's helplessness, fear, and weakness in different situations and their limitations and blind spots. When students can see the context behind the incident, it is an essential humanistic ability and the basis of empathy or compassion. When students can see the context behind the incident, it is an essential humanistic ability and the basis of empathy or compassion.

In addition, we also arrange "life story sharing by care recipients" and "caregivers' experiences in practicing humanistic care." Because the narration and the story have the power of moving resonance, nursing students recognize the value of people through storytelling. Therefore, with a series of storytelling learning, international volunteers are invited to share their personal life beliefs and traveler stories of international service. Through the videos and photos of the stories, the students realize that the work of helping others can range from clinical work to cross-border. This sharing activated the enthusiasm and confidence of the students, and it turns out that the field of nursing work can be a humanistic care action without borders.

At the end of the course, the nursing students reviewed their clinical experience, reflected on their humanistic care, and explored their understanding of humanistic care; to think about how to practice humanistic care, make the nursing process more humane, give full play to the spirit of humanistic care, and make nursing work an art of caring for people. In the reflection on the process of the teaching plan, nursing students mentioned their worries about the future practice environment, and burnout is also a notable problem. Nurses need to be respected and cared for, considering their limitations and vulnerabilities. How the humanistic quality becomes a nutrient and turns around to nourish nurses, enrich each other's life, become an internal motivation, or plant humanistic seeds in the heart, is a direction worth exploring in the future. It is also an essential purpose of this teaching plan design. We believe that "putting yourself in the shoes" in the teaching program of nursing humanities is not a realistic and achievable goal; just as it is difficult for us to understand the world of "autistic" patients, we must infer the patient's feelings from their reactions. Only through teaching program design, good use of media materials, dialog and discussion, and experience reflection, nursing students can be trained to have multiple thinking and deep awareness and be prepared for their future careers. This is the feasible teaching plan for the nursing humanities course.

6. Nursing professional development trends and humanistic education

Nursing professional development has been influenced by the specialization and institutionalization of the health care system. With the division of medical specialties, patient care has become oriented to disease diagnosis and biomedical treatment. Professional care is often provided according to physician order, neglecting that human beings not only have bodies but also minds and spirits. The patient care often generalizes and decontextualizes the essence of the nursing profession.

To counterbalance this situation, nursing professional development should place more emphasis on humanistic education. Nursing professors must have humanistic qualities, including tolerance, appreciation, and a respectful and caring attitude.

The key to the development of nursing students' humanistic care ability is teachers possessing the competence to implement humanities education in their own instruction. Therefore, the key to the success or failure of humanities education is ensuring, through the professional development process, that nursing professors have this competence [47]. Only professional teachers that have humanistic qualities and practice the essence of nursing humanities can serve as role models, naturally influencing their students as they implement humanistic care in clinical practice [19].

Ideal humanities education teachers would have both professional nursing as well as humanities and social sciences training. The lack of teachers with this training creates a challenge for nursing professional development. The authors suggest that humanities and professional teachers should work together to open nursing courses. Teachers should be able to identify with humanistic qualities, teaching as much by example as by through their words, allowing students to recognize the necessity of humanistic literacy [48].

To reiterate, promotion of humanities education and the cultivation of humanities teachers must be achieved in order to improve the humanistic cultivation of nursing staff. This is the key element that must be implemented in the process of nursing professional development [3].

7. Conclusion

A humanistic education in the nursing profession will allow nursing students to provide an affective experience of humanity, care, and esthetic appreciation, to develop a broader perspective, to cultivate insight, to understand and feel the unique experience of patients, and to look at problems from multiple perspectives, especially in complex situations. The challenge of today's nursing education is using multiple teaching strategies to improve humanistic cultivation in the humanities education in the nursing profession. We recommend actively advocating the use of 6E as a teaching strategy framework to promote humanistic nursing education and integrating the experience of literature and artistic esthetics to enhance the affective experience of nursing staff at the perceptual level. At the same time, through self-awareness and reflection, nursing staff can strengthen deep empathy and keen observation ability, improve humanistic quality, and practice the humanistic spirit in professional nursing, which promotes the nursing process to be more humane.

Conflict of interest

The author declares no conflicts of interest.

Funding

These researches were funded by the Taiwan National Science Council (Grant Number NSC99-2511-S-255-001-MY2, NSC102-2511-S-255-004-MY2) and Chang Gung Memorial Hospital.

The data that support the findings of these studies are available on request from the Principal Investigator, M.-Y.Y.

The data are not publicly available due to their containing information that could compromise the privacy of research participants.

Author details

Mei-Yu Yeh
Department of Nursing, Kang Ning University, Taipei City, Taiwan, Republic of China

*Address all correspondence to: yehdiana8@gmail.com

References

[1] Amit P. 5 predictions for how technology will transform healthcare in 2022... and beyond. 2022. Available from: https://medcitynews.com/2022/01/5-predictions-for-how-technology-will-transform-healthcare-in-2022-and-beyond/ [Accessed: August 20, 2022]

[2] Huang CC. Exploration of General Education in College and University: The Enlightenment from Taiwan Experiences. Taipei City, Taiwan, ROC: Chinese Association for General Education; 2009. p. 256

[3] Yeh MY, Liao PC, Lu CF, Lin HC, Sung SC, Lo WT, et al. Nursing and Humanities. 1st ed. Taipei: Wu-Nan; 2018. p. 226 (Chinese)

[4] Miles A, Mezzich JE. Mint: The care of the patient and the soul of the clinic: Person-centered medicine as an emergent model of modern clinical practice. International Journal of Person Centered Medicine. 2011;**1**:207-222 (Chinese)

[5] Huang KY. Mint: Put the humanities back to medical curriculum. The Journal of General Education. 1996;**3**:1-16 (Chinese)

[6] Yeh MY, Lee S. Mint: The Spirit of humanism should Be cultivated in the nursing profession. The Journal of Nursing. 2011;**58**:12-16

[7] Peng HS. Mint: Concepts and reflection of humanity education: A perspective from educational history. Newsletter for Teaching the Humanities and Social Sciences. 2001;**12**:155-177 (Chinese)

[8] Tai MCT. Mint: The challenge of medical humanities. Formosan Journal of Medicine. 2007;**11**:163-166 (Chinese)

[9] Marnocha S, Marnocha M. Mint: Windows open: Humanities teaching during undergraduate clinical experiences. The Journal of Nursing Education. 2007;**46**:518-521

[10] Pardue KT. Mint: Blending aesthetics and empirics: Teaching health assessment in an art gallery. The Journal of Nursing Education. 2005;**44**:334-337

[11] Tsui HC, Ho MJ. Mint: The evolution of medical humanities education in Taiwan: Qualitative analysis by in-depth interviews. Journal of Medical Education. 2008;**12**:133-141 (Chinese)

[12] Chiang HH. Mint: Constructing ethical approaches through nursing practice. The Journal of Nursing. 2002;**49**:20-24 (Chinese)

[13] Chang HJ. Mint: Medical history and medical humanity education. Formosan Journal of Medicine. 2007;**11**:167-170 (Chinese)

[14] Tai MCT. Mint: Medical humanity and medical education. Chung Shan Medical Journal. 2000;**11**:1-6 (Chinese)

[15] Lazenby M. Mint: On the humanities of nursing. Nursing Outlook. 2013;**61**:9-14

[16] Wu LC, Yang YO. Mint: Humanity and clinical nursing. Veterans General Hospital Nursing. 2011;**28**:104-110 (Chinese)

[17] Dellasega C, Milone-Nuzzo P, Curci KM, Ballard JO, Kirch DG. Mint: The humanities interface of nursing and medicine. Journal of Professional Nursing. 2007;**23**:174-179

[18] Watson J. Mint: What, may I ask is happening to nursing knowledge

and professional practices? What is nursing thinking at this turn in human history? Journal of Clinical Nursing. 2005;**14**:913-914

[19] Shiau SJ, Chiang YT, Huang YC, Chiu PR, Feng RF, Heh SC, et al. Mint: The life cultivation of nursing education touched by care concern and compassion. Journal of Medical Education. 2006;**10**:1-7 (Chinese)

[20] Calman KC. Mint: The arts and humanities in health and medicine. Royal Institute Public Health. 2005;**119**:958-959

[21] Donohoe M, Danielson S. Mint: A community-based approach to the medical humanities. Medical Education. 2004;**38**:204-217

[22] Einstein A. Mint: Medicine, the arts, and the humanities. Lancet. 2003;**362**:93-94

[23] Gull ES. Mint: Embedding the humanities into medical education. Medical Education. 2005;**39**:235-236

[24] Lin HJ, Wang SY, Lai CS, Lin YC. Mint: Narrative medical ethics curriculum the experience from Kaohsiung Medical University. Journal of Medical Education. 2010;**14**:22-31 (Chinese)

[25] Bleakley A, Marshall R. Mint: Can the science of communication inform the art of the medical humanities? Medical Education. 2013;**47**:126-133

[26] Polson GR, Farmer SE. Mint: Integrating the humanities in the education of health professionals: Implications for search and retrieval of information. Nurse Education in Practice. 2002;**2**:49-54

[27] Pei JK. Mint: The general education of the medical humanities: A perspective of linguistics and medical history. Journal of the Chinese for General Education. 2005;**7**:1-16

[28] Chou CC, Suen LJ, Lin YC. Mint: Humanity education in nursing. The Journal of Nursing. 2007;**54**:29-34

[29] Yeh MY. Faculty developmental program in nursing humanities education. In: Proceedings of the National Science Council Conference on Medical Education. Taipei, National Science Council; 2015

[30] Ryan K. The six E's of character education. At Boston University School of Education. [Internet] 2009. Available from: http://www.bu.edu/sed/caec/files/6E.htm [Accessed: December 30, 2009]

[31] Darbyshire P. Mint: Understanding caring through arts and humanities: A medical/nursing humanities approach to promoting alterative experiences of thinking and learning. Journal of Advanced Nursing. 1995;**19**:856-863

[32] Chiang HH, Shu BC. Mint: Ethical skills in the care of the self. The Journal of Nursing. 2006;**53**:20-24

[33] Ho MJ. Mint: Literature and medicine: Examples of humanity education in medicine. Chung-Wai Literary Monthly. 2003;**31**:10-25

[34] Moyle W, Barnard A, Turner C. Mint: The humanities and nursing: Using popular literature as a means of understanding human experience. Journal of Advanced Nursing. 1995;**21**:960-964

[35] Huang CY, Wang LC, Ho MJ. Mint: Special report on a faculty development workshop concerning narrative medicine. Journal of Medical Education. 2010;**14**:54-61 (Chinese)

[36] Liu JS, Kho WS, Lin YS, Chang WY. Mint: A search of the creative practice for an indigenous medical humanities education: A project of narrative and writing of illness from the perspectives of medical students and patients. Formosan J Medical Humanities. 2003;**4**:84-107 (Chinese)

[37] Kuo YL, Lee JT, Yeh MY. Intergenerational narrative learning to bridge the generation gap in humanistic care nursing education. Healthcare. 2021;**29**:1291. DOI: 10.3390/healthcare9101291. PMID: 34682971; PMCID: PMC8535847

[38] Walsh M. Narrative pedagogy and simulation: Future directions for nursing education. Nurse Education in Practice. 2011;**11**(3):216-219

[39] Bleakley A, Marshall R. Can the science of communication inform the art of the medical humanities? Medical Education. 2013;**47**(2):126-133

[40] Marnocha S, Marnocha M. Windows open: Humanities teaching during undergraduate clinical experiences. The Journal of Nursing Education. 2007;**46**(11):518-521

[41] Wang CC, Geale SK. The power of story: Narrative inquiry as a methodology in nursing research. IJNSS. 2015;**2**(2):195-198

[42] Earle V, Myrick F. Nursing pedagogy and the intergenerational discourse. The Journal of Nursing Education. 2009;**48**:624-630. DOI: 10.3928/01484834-20090716-08

[43] Chen SYC. Learning process and effects of incorporating intergenerational learning in a social gerontology course. Journal of Research in Education Sciences. 2014;**59**:1-28. DOI: 10.6209/JORIES.2014.59(3).01 (Chinese)

[44] Gutheil IA, Chernesky RH, Sherratt ML. Influencing student attitudes toward older adults: Results of a service-learning collaboration. Educational Gerontology. 2006;**32**(9):771-784

[45] Meshel DS, McGlynn RP. Intergenerational contact, attitudes, and stereotypes of adolescents and older people. Educational Gerontology. 2004;**30**(6):457-479

[46] Lazenby M. On the humanities of nursing. Nursing Outlook. 2013;**61**(1):9-14

[47] Wang SY. Truthful concepts of general education: Program of medical humanities curriculum. The Journal of General Education. 2006;**1**:33-48 (Chinese)

[48] Kao MY, Lue BH, Chuu LI. The practices and dilemmas of medical humanities curriculum in Taiwan. Journal of Medical Education. 2004;**8**(4):392-403 (Chinese)

Chapter 5

Enhancement of Learning Abilities of Student Nurses: Teaching and Learning Strategies

Beryl Juliet Sam

Abstract

The modern era poses a great challenge for students pursuing the baccalaureate program in nursing sciences. The Program requires rigorous hours of learning and clinical exposure. Nursing has now moved into a competency-based curriculum. The global demand for nurses is expected to rise to 9 million in the 2030. Hence, the profession needs a lot of dedicated and inspired minds with sacrifice and accountability. Students in general have a variety of learning styles that aids their learning process. This chapter focusses on the various strategies that nurse educators and faculty should adopt, to help students cope with the demands of the profession. There are a variety of strategies that can be used, however, each one has its own pros and cons. Nursing curriculum is centered on producing professionals who are committed to caring real-life clients. It's the duty of nurse leaders, managers and educationists in sculpting young minds to work towards making a significant difference in the lives of others.

Keywords: enhancement, learning abilities, learning strategies, teaching strategies, nursing students

1. Introduction

Nursing is one of the most noble professions in the world. "A nurse is one who opens the eyes of a newborn baby and closes the eyes of the dying". The modern day students need a lot of innovative technologies to enhance their learning. They also have to be exposed to interesting learning strategies that faculty must provide. The competency-based curriculum demands expertise in both the cognitive and psychomotor domains. This chapter will deal with various contemporary methods of teaching and learning.

A study by Gundus and Ozcan on the learning styles of Learning styles of students from different cultures and studying in Near East University found that, cultures of the students affect their learning styles. Arabic students learn more actively than Turkish and Cypriot students. Thus, each student learns in a different way, and to address these learning styles, teachers should use a variety of teaching styles [1].

Students are found to be very passive and disinterested during the traditional teaching methods. There has to be an inclusion of different problem based learning methods that provokes the thought process of students. Nurses are expected to practice in varied settings, and hence the need for equipping them with adequate knowledge to adapt to any situation is the need of the hour [2] Heidgerken explains the fact that, it is not enough if a faculty in nursing poses mere knowledge to teach nursing curriculum to students. They need to possess specialized skills to teach in a variety of settings. Nurses play different roles of caregiving, educating, advocating, and carrying out research. Hence, faculty members should enable the student to have adequate exposure to be effectively equipped to play all these roles [3].

Students also need an exciting experience to learn concepts so that they do not feel bored with traditional system of learning. It is necessary for faculty to update to the latest technology to cater to students in the contemporary era. The teaching process prepares the student nurse to play all the roles that the society expects of her as a full-fledged nurse. Hence, the learning process should be a rigorous period of inculcating necessary skills through several methods.

2. Innovative teaching methods in the nursing curriculum

A wide range of teaching methods are being used by nursing faculty. A few of them will be discussed in this chapter. Some of them are, Flipped Learning, Edpuzzle, Simulation, Virtual Patient Learning, Self-Directed Learning, Problem based learning, Team based Learning and Inter professional education. Innovative approaches will help increase the effectiveness and efficiency of the entire clinical nursing education system that the program offers [4].

2.1 Flipped classroom learning

Flipped learning is new to most students, and it generally takes time to adjust to the pedagogy. Five factors are thought to affect a student's readiness for the flipped classroom. They are perceptions of workload, attitude towards active learning, relevant educational experience, metacognitive skills, and comfort with technology. To help all students benefit from flipped learning at the earliest stages of the class, an orientation is proposed that reduces the potential negative impact of each of these factors. Special advice is provided for first-year students, as they are inexperienced with flipped learning. Freshmen are still adapting to University life. So, there may be low-performing students who may need extra support to fully benefit from the pedagogy [5].

Barbour and Schuessler stated that, though clinical and healthcare settings have grown in complexity over the last several years, the way we educate nursing students remains unchanged. This transformation places a demand on nursing faculty to shift their traditional teaching system to more innovative methods like Flipped Classroom Method (FCM). FCM enhances critical thinking skills of students and enables them to apply this knowledge received outside the class to real-world scenarios and problems within the class [6].

A research on perception of 240 student nurses' on flipped classroom showed a positive attitude towards this type of learning. The use of video and moodle, showed that they had a positive attitude towards FCM. There was also a strong correlation on perceptions of motivation, self engagement, enhanced and effective learning. The attitudes of low achievers was much more positive as compared to high achievers [7]. The FCM and the virtual experience that students gain out of it helps students learn what cannot be taught through a mere lecture in the physical classroom [8]. Akcayır and Akcayır stated that the challenges faced by students while learning out of the class improved their learning process [9]. FCM uses a system designed with lectures that are pre-recorded, short quizzes and activities. They help increase the motivation level of students and cultivates a better learning environment [10].

The FCM is a best example of a learner-centered approach and it is beneficial for both the student and the faculty when compared to traditional lecture methods [11]. The current didactic teaching method does not help nursing students to efficiently apply their theoretical knowledge to clinical situations. The revolution needed in nursing education in the contemporary era poses a need where, educational methods must be designed to apply skills to problem solve [12]. The flipped classroom (FC), was considered to be a novel method of teaching that emphasized Self Directed Learning (SDL) and critical thinking among student nurses in China [13].

A study on the comparison of critical thinking among Second year Iranian nursing students who had traditional vs. flipped classroom learning showed that, those exposed to FC had significant positive effects on their critical thinking when compared to the other group [14]. A mixed methods research was done on the perception of FCL and its impact of learning among undergraduate nursing students from three universities in Sri Lanka. Findings showed that, students perceived it to be highly beneficial and promising [15].

2.2 Edpuzzle

One of the most interesting methods by which students can be attracted to learn concepts in an easy way with their full involvement is edpuzzle. Introducing edpuzzle to students prior to their lab sessions helped in increasing student learning in biochemistry course as reported in a study [16]. This application helps students maximize their learning outcomes while giving teachers an insight into the areas that students perceive as difficult. It will also allow the faculty to readdress the same in the classroom [17].

The current pandemic Covid-19 posed a threat to the traditional teaching methods in nursing education. However, it was augmented with online modules and other applications that enabled students graduate with transformations in the nursing curriculum. The content that must be studied in the classroom was supplemented with youtube educational videos, virtual platforms and other online material. Edpuzzle serves as an interactive as well as an excellent educative online material that helped nurse educators enhance learning [18].

2.3 Simulation

Simulation is a method that involves teaching students by using case scenarios and creating a realistic learning experience. High fidelity simulation is a growing teaching method and has changed to include highly sophisticated and interactive simulators which helps students learn in a non-threatening environment [2].

Students pursuing health care professions are expected to deal with real patients. They often feel very scared, threatened and inadequate when it comes to applying or re-demonstrating clinical skills. Simulation can be explained as an artificially created or man-made replication by which students can learn in order to acquire the necessary clinical skills. They can be manikins or equipment that will enable students to practice on several times, without the fear of harming or endangering the life of the patient. It also helps learners gain expertise and competence [19].

Health science faculty use this as an effective strategy for teaching, learning and training as it gives a near to normal experience for students [20]. Owing to the Covid-19 pandemic, it was practically impossible for learners to gain adequate clinical learning exposure. The simulation labs serve as an atmosphere of actual client centered learning. Many students have a high level of cognition which helps them grasp concepts at a satisfying level. However, when it comes to putting their knowledge into practice, they find it difficult to carryout techniques and demonstrate appropriate clinical skills and manual dexterity [21].

A study regarding Simulation based Learning on Clinical decision making and Communication skills among 88 student nurses revealed that, learning using the SBAR tool helped in precise clinical decision making and professional communication which showed significance at p = <.0001 level [22]. A study on perceptions of Simulation Based Learning (SBL) among students pursuing medicine had majority (90.7%) reporting that, SBL helped in development of their clinical skills. Findings also revealed that the perceptions were higher among female students than males [23].

A study on supporting students through eLearning showed promising results regarding simulation based learning as it helps students learn in a safe and non-threatening environment without the fear of harming patients. The results also showed enhanced performance, better grades and self efficacy in carrying out nursing procedures [24].

2.4 Virtual patient learning

Virtual Patient cases (VP cases) promote learning, teaching, and assessment of clinical reasoning and can stimulate and motivate active learning experiences in nursing education [25]. A study was conducted among 45 first-year and 31 third-year undergraduate nursing students using a case study method with focus groups and individual interviews with the aim of exploring the experience of interaction with a virtual patient in order to develop non-technical skills. Findings indicated that, students at different levels interacted differently with the virtual patients. Four themes were identified in the data (i.e.) how the virtual patients enabled learning non-technical skills, learning regarding the virtual patient encounter, changing the way students perceive practice and the potential limitations to learning [26].

Prelicensure baccalaureate nursing students' perceptions and experiences of using virtual simulation as an alternative to clinical practice during the (COVID-19) pandemic was assessed in South Korea. Findings showed that, Virtual simulation might help pre-licensure nursing students feel more competent and confident [27]. VP cases provided support in translating theoretical knowledge into clinical reasoning, and they facilitated the application of theory in practice and encouraged students to use their clinical reasoning. It also enabled self-evaluation, which was a motivating force and increased awareness of their abilities for clinical reasoning. Learning experiences from VP cases seem to be applicable in higher education and useful in enabling nursing students to apply theory in their clinical practice [28].

A quasi experimental study was carried out to evaluate the effectiveness of VPL on social learning among 40 senior nursing students with 20 in the intervention group and 20 in the non-intervention group. Study results showed that Virtual patients made the learning process more enjoyable and also enhanced the learning of students.

In addition to it, VPL also proved to be effective in improving the communication skills of students [29].

2.5 Self directed learning

Self directed learning (SDL) is another method that enables the nursing student to use his/her critical thinking skills and also increases independence and leads students towards professional competence. An experimental study on SDL with blended learning was carried out among 91 students where the study group and control group had 44 and 47 participants respectively. The intervention group was trained using an SDL program with blended coaching. Those in the experimental group showed a highly significant improvement and were competent in implementation of SDL ($F(1,89) = 4.27$, $p = 0.039$). They were also found to have a higher satisfaction with clinical practice at the bedside ($t(89) = 3.10$, $p = 0.003$) compared with those in the non-intervention group. Nursing faculty believe that this method increases the students' assertiveness, accountability and makes them develop a sense of responsibility that they need to exercise in their career [30].

A cross sectional comparative study examined the extent of self-directed learning abilities among 1746 nursing students and its possible factors in six European countries. Findings revealed that, the overall SDL abilities were high among students from all countries with statistically significant differences between the countries. It was found that, Spanish nursing students reported the highest level of SDL abilities while students from the Czech Republic reported the lowest. Higher level of self-directed learning abilities was related to several factors, particularly with self-assessed level of competence and geographical location [31].

A study explored the effect of PBL on 12 Iranian students pursuing Masters program in Nursing. The findings indicated that, the students adopted various methods of different SDL for excelling in academics. They also had a lot of perseverance and curiosity that played an important role in their SDL in challenging areas [32].

The readiness for SDL along with learning styles was explored using a cross sectional study among 236 Omani student nurses. Findings showed a low level of SDL and also a negative association between the learning styles and SDL [33]. Students in the health professions education have very limited time to learn vast curriculum and syllabi in the classroom. Hence it is essential that they are encouraged and guided to SDL outside their classrooms. Majority of students reported that, a good lecture led them to SDL [34]. Nursing is a profession in which lifelong learning has to take place. SDL is a very valuable skill that will enable nursing students to adopt SDL and develop these skills. Totally 229 student nurses from South-West Nigeria participated in a study on SDL. The pretest knowledge was assessed followed by 6 weeks interaction by SDL on selected topics in Adult health nursing. A post test was carried out at the end of 6 weeks. The findings revealed a significant improvement in knowledge scores between the pre and post test [35].

A study among 800 student nurses on the associations between SDL and professional nursing values revealed that, male nursing students had higher levels of self-directed learning [36]. Wong, Tang and Chang in their systematic review of 18 studies on SDL reported that, SDL must be encouraged in health professions education because it nurtures self-motivation among students and promotes liability to their own learning. Further more, it is crucial to fostering collaborative skills for multi-disciplinary practice in the contemporary era [37].

2.6 Problem based learning

Problem Based Learning (PBL) is yet another method that promotes teaching and learning among nursing professionals. Nursing curricula is aimed at preparing professionals to deal efficiently with any crisis that they may encounter in patient care and in managing daily challenges as a bedside nurse, patient educator or nurse administrator. Hence problem based strategy which promotes critical thinking is the need of the hour in order to keep in pace and be both confident and competent [38]. Crawford in his article on web-based PBL stated that, PBL is a technique used to discuss clinical case scenarios and it enables students to think deeply towards problem solving, thereby making them aware of the several options and also creating more accountability and responsibility [39].

Critical thinking, problem-solving, and SDL of 90 first year nursing students in two universities receiving PBL vs. traditional lecture, was carried out in South Korea. One group received PBL while the others were given traditional lectures. An initial pretest was given and a post test was done after 16 weeks on aspects like critical thinking, problem-solving, and self-directed learning abilities. There was a significant positive correlation between both groups. The students in the PBL group had an overall improvement across all abilities measured, while students in the traditional lecture group showed a decreased problem-solving ability and lowered levels of self-directed learning [40].

2.7 Electronic learning

When students are directed to use eLearning in the right way, it can maximize the effects and help in enhancement of knowledge [41]. There is a huge challenge for nursing faculty as they impart education and skills to student nurses. The nursing curriculum is seeking to produce young minds with in-depth knowledge and competence while being equipped with decision making skills [42].

The Covid-19 pandemic posed a threat to on-site learning. A lot of e-learning took place without compromise on nursing education. The satisfaction of nursing students and the perceived barriers to online learning was studied among 219 nursing students. Results revealed that, majority (67.6%) were extremely satisfied with e-learning. Among the perceived barriers which restricted online learning, the highest was a low pitched voice and clarity of language (2.16 ± 0.593). The biological/physical barriers were vision related problems (2.43 ± 0.613) and network issues (2.26 ± 0.534). There was a significant association between the age of nursing students with the extent of satisfaction regarding online learning [43].

Web based learning has assisted students to a great extent. Nowadays the use of electronic learning has become unquestionable among students in the health professions education. The advancement and utilization of information technology even when all educational institutions were shut during the pandemic brought a solution and enhanced uninterrupted learning. An online survey on web based learning among 490 nursing students revealed that, only 34% of them found that e learning was as effective as face to face learning. More than half (58.9%) of them had a favorable attitude towards e-learning. Majority (81.7%) of them had issues with internet connections followed by technical issues (65.5%). If these barriers can be reduced, online learning will be the best method for educating nursing students [44]. An integrative review on attitudes of nursing students towards learning using the mobile specified that, majority of nursing students have a positive attitude and willingness towards mobile learning, but practically, the actual use rate was low. This was thought to be due to unstable network connectivity and technical problems [45].

2.8 InterProfessional education

Interprofessional education (IPE) is an emerging method where team based learning takes place among students from various health related professions. It enables students to learn together and also to learn from each other. A planned IPE program was offered to students from two universities in Hong Kong. Students who belonged to various healthcare disciplines like medicine, nursing, pharmacy, biomedical science, and Chinese medicine programs were included in the study. Anonymous questionnaires were given to 40 nursing students in order to gauge their IPE experience. There was a statistically significant improvement in the knowledge level ($p < 0.001$), attitude towards readiness for IPE, team based learning, and perceived group efficacy ($p < 0.001$) [46].

A mixed method design was used to measure the interprofessional competencies and attitudes among students pursuing health professions education on virtual patient cases. Students participated and worked together as a team in developing virtual case based patient learning modules on family planning. The changes in perception of students belonging to various health care professions was assessed before and after the project work. Results revealed a statistically significant increase in the students' self-assessment competency scores. An improvement in interprofessional collaboration skills was observed among students from various disciplines at the end of the study [47].

IPE is thought to advance learning among students in the health professions and also promote the quality of health care delivery [48]. When students from various health professions meet and work together on a case, it allows collaboration of health care. It involves a lot of thought processes and helps cater to the needs of clients. IPE enables knowledge and skills that are essential for collaborative working to be learnt [49].

2.9 Team based learning

One of the most innovative strategy that nursing faculty can plan for their students is Team based learning (TBL). It helps in imparting knowledge and skills that students will find easy to understand. This could prove to be very effective because it is very well structured, thus enhancing a student-friendly learning environment [50].

A study helped determine the factors that influenced satisfaction of nursing students in regards to Team based Learning (TBL) in Korea. Team-based learning sessions consisting of preparation, readiness assurance, and application were given to a cohort of 139 second year nursing students in 2010 and 263 students in 2011 respectively. At the end of the learning sessions, participants completed a self-administered questionnaire regarding their learning experience. Nursing students were generally satisfied with team-based learning. Multiple regression analysis revealed that the learning process significantly affected learner satisfaction compared to pre-assignment, course content, peer evaluation, and team activity [51].

A study was undertaken in order to apply TBL in four nursing courses and to assess its effect on the learning outcomes and behaviors among 387 Registered Nurse-Bachelor of Science in Nursing students (RNBSN) and Bachelor of Science in Nursing

(BSN) students at a University in Taiwan. Medical Surgical nursing, Obstetrics and Pediatric nursing, Public health nursing, and Adult nursing were the four courses chosen for the study. Results revealed that the TBL significantly improved the learning behaviors of students in both the nursing programs, including self involvement in the classroom ($p < .001$) and SDL ($p < .001$). The study concluded that TBL generally improves academic performance and learning among students [52].

TBL is considered to be one of the most effective method of small group learning where the student nurse is benefitted to a great extent. The TBL can be a faculty led learning experience with a student – faculty ratio as less as 7:1 without comprise on the course delivery in a group even as large as 200:1. A study that sought to assess the efficacy of TBL in regards to involvement and engagement of students in the process, found it to be very effective [53].

A study was conducted on the impact of TBL on first year undergraduate nursing students in relation to their knowledge, application and attitude on integration of concepts learnt in the process. Majority of students (70%) reported an increase in knowledge, skills and satisfaction in working together as a team [54]. The effect of TBL on the critical thinking, problem solving ability and SDL of students was carried out among 167 junior student nurses working with clients suffering from disorders of the respiratory system. The study design was a one-group pretest-posttest design. The students had TBL sessions for 2 hours a week for a period of six weeks. Findings showed a significant improvement in critical thinking disposition ($t = 5.02$, $p < .001$), problem solving ability ($t = -6.04$, $p < .001$), and self-directed learning ($t = 5.96$, $p < .001$). There was a significant positive correlation among problem solving ability, critical thinking skills and SDL among the undergraduate students [55].

3. Conclusion

This chapter has provided a brief description of the various teaching learning strategies in nursing education. With rapid advancements in the field of science and technology, nursing is a profession where, life long learning has to take place in order to stay updated. This places a demand on student nurses to widen their horizon of learning than getting self satisfied with what is only taught in the classroom [28]. In a systematic review [55], the authors rightly pointed out that, life long learning strategies must be incorporated in the nursing profession as it will not only enhance the overall knowledge, skills and core competencies of a nurse; but will directly lead to improved quality of patient care. All nurse educators and faculty must deem it the need of the hour to enable students to develop a positive attitude towards life long learning and also use a solid evidence-base to implement it. Nurse leaders who are responsible for planning the nursing curriculum should also place emphasis on the need for change in the syllabi if required.

Acknowledgements

The author wishes to thank Intech Open publishers for the opportunity and financial support rendered to publish this chapter. A special note of thanks to friends and family for their love and support in successful completion of this chapter. No funding was received for publishing this work.

Conflict of interest

The author declares no conflict of interest.

Author details

Beryl Juliet Sam
College of Nursing, Gulf Medical University, Ajman, UAE

*Address all correspondence to: beryljsam@gmail.com

References

[1] Gunduz N, Ozcan D. Learning styles of students from different cultures and studying in near east university. Procedia - Social and Behavioral Sciences. 2010;**9**:5-10. DOI: 10.1016/j.sbspro.2010.12.107

[2] Korukcua O, Kukulu K. Innovation in nursing education. Procedia Social and Behavioral Sciences. 2010;**9**:369-372

[3] Heidgerken LE. Teaching and Learning in Schools of Nursing-Principles and Methods. 3rd ed. India: Konark Publishers International; 2012

[4] Niederhauser V, Schoessler M, Gubrud-Howe PM, Magnussen L, Codier E. Creating innovative models of clinical nursing education. The Journal of Nursing Education. 2012;**51**(11):603-608. DOI: 10.3928/01484834-20121011-02

[5] Roehling PV. Flipping the College Classroom. 2018. DOI: 10.1007/978-3-319-69392-7

[6] Barbour C, Schuessler JB. A preliminary framework to guide implementation of the flipped classroom method in nursing education. Nurse Education in Practice. 2019;**34**:36-42. DOI: 10.1016/j.nepr.2018.11.001

[7] Nouri J. The flipped classroom: For active, effective and increased learning – Especially for low achievers. International Journal of Educational Technology in Higher Education. 2016;**13**:33. DOI: 10.1186/s41239-016-0032-z

[8] Roehling PV. Introduction to flipped learning. In: Flipping the College Classroom. Cham: Palgrave Pivot; 2018. DOI: 10.1007/978-3-319-69392-7_1

[9] Akcayır G, Akcayır M. The flipped classroom: A review of its advantages and challenges. Computers & Education. 2018;**126**:334-345. DOI: 10.1016/j.compedu.2018.07.021

[10] Awidi IT, Paynter M. The impact of a flipped classroom approach on student learning experience. Computers & Education. 2019;**128**:269-283. DOI: 10.1016/j.compedu.2018.09.013

[11] Gilboy MB, Heinerichs S, Pazzaglia G. Enhancing student engagement using the flipped classroom. Journal of Nutrition Education and Behavior. 2015;**47**(1):109-114. DOI: 10.1016/j.jneb.2014.08.008

[12] Betihavas V, Bridgman H, Kornhaber R, Cross M. The evidence for 'flipping out': A systematic review of the flipped classroom in nursing education. Nurse Education Today. 2016;**38**:15-21. DOI: 10.1016/j.nedt.2015.12.010

[13] Li BZ, Cao NW, Ren CX, Chu XJ, Zhou HY, et al. Flipped classroom improves nursing students' theoretical learning in China: A meta-analysis, Flipped classroom improves nursing students' theoretical learning in China: A meta-analysis. PLoS One. 2020;**15**(8):e0237926

[14] Dehghanzadeha S, Jafaraghaeeb F. Comparing the effects of traditional lecture and flipped classroom on nursing students' critical thinking disposition: A quasi-experimental study. Nurse Education Today. 2018;**71**:151-156. DOI: 10.1016/j.nedt.2018.09.027

[15] Youhasan P, Chen Y, Lyndon M, Henning MA. Assess the feasibility of flipped classroom pedagogy in undergraduate nursing education in Sri

Lanka: A mixed-methods study. PLoS One. 2021;**16**(11):e0259003. DOI: 10.1371/journal.pone.0259003

[16] Shelby SJ, Fralish ZD. Using Edpuzzle to improve student experience and performance in the biochemistry laboratory. Biochemistry and Molecular Biology Education. 2021;**49**:529-534

[17] Littlefield and Amber. Increasing cognitive thinking skills with Edpuzzle. Nurse Educator. 2019;**44**(2):78

[18] de Tantillo L, Christopher R. Transforming graduate nursing education during an era of social distancing: Tools from the field. Nurse Education Today. 2020;**92**:104472. DOI: 10.1016/j.nedt.2020.104472 Epub 2020 May 29

[19] Al-Elq AH. Simulation-based medical teaching, and learning. Journal of Family and Community Medicine. 2010;**17**(1):35-40. DOI: 10.4103/1319-1683.68787

[20] Agha S, Alhamrani A, Khan M. Satisfaction of medical students with simulation-based learning. Saudi Medical Journal. 2015;**36**:731-736. DOI: 10.15537%2Fsmj.2015.6.1150

[21] Alinier G, Hunt B, Gordon R, Harwood C. Effectiveness of intermediate–fidelity simulation training technology in undergraduate nursing education. Journal of Advanced Nursing. 2006;**54**:359-369. DOI: 10.1111/j.1365-2648.2006.03810.x

[22] Oh H. Effects of simulation learning using SBAR on clinical judgement and communication skills in undergraduate nursing students. International Journal of Contents. 2021;**17**(3):30-37. ISSN: 1738-6764, eISSN: 2093-7504

[23] Docherty C, Hoy D, Topp H. Kathryn Trinder, eLearning techniques supporting problem based learning in clinical simulation. International Journal of Medical Informatics. 2005;**74**(7-8):527-533. DOI: 10.1016/j.ijmedinf.2005.03.009

[24] Ellaway R, Poulton T, Fors U, McGee JB, Albright S. Building a virtual patient is common. Medical Teacher. 2008;**30**(2):170-174. DOI: 10.1080/01421590701874074

[25] Kononowicz AA, Zary N, Edelbring S, Corral J, Hege I. Virtual patients—What are we talking about? A framework to classify the meanings of the term in healthcare education. BMC Medical Education. 2015;**15**(1):1-11. DOI: 10.1186/s12909-015-0296-3

[26] Goldsworthy S, Muir N, Baron S, Button D, Goodhand K, Hunter S, et al. The impact of virtual simulation on the recognition and response to the rapidly deteriorating patient among undergraduate nursing students. Nurse Education Today. 2022;**110**:105264. DOI: 10.1016/j.nedt.2021.105264

[27] Forsberg E, Backlund B, Telhede EH, Karlsson S. Virtual patient cases for active student participation in nursing education —Students' learning experiences. Creative Education. 2019;**10**(7):1475-1491

[28] Hwang GJ, Chang CY, Ogata H. The effectiveness of the virtual patient-based social learning approach in undergraduate nursing education: A quasi-experimental study. Nurse Education Today. 2022;**108**:105164. DOI: 10.1016/j.nedt.2021.105164 Epub 2021 Oct 4

[29] Noh GO, Kim D. Effectiveness of a self-directed learning program using blended coaching among nursing students in clinical practice: A quasi-experimental research design. BMC

Medical Education. 2019;**19**:225. DOI: 10.1186/s12909-019-1672-1

[30] Visiers-Jiménez L, Palese A, Brugnolli A, Cadorin L, Salminen L, Leino-Kilpi H, et al. Nursing students' self-directed learning abilities and related factors at graduation: A multi-country cross-sectional study. Nursing Open. 2022;**9**(3):1688-1699. DOI: 10.1002/nop2.1193 Epub 2022 Feb 13

[31] Shirazi F, Sharif F, Molazem Z, Alborzi M. Dynamics of self-directed learning in m.Sc. Nursing students: A qualitative research. Journal of Advances in Medical Education & Professionalism. 2017;**5**(1):33-41

[32] Ballad CAC, Labrague LJ, Cayaban ARR, Turingan OM, Al Balushi SM. Self-directed learning readiness and learning styles among Omani nursing students: Implications for online learning during the COVID-19 pandemic. Nursing Forum. 2022;**57**(1):94-103. DOI: 10.1111/nuf.12664 Epub 2021 Oct 21

[33] Business Bliss Consultants FZE. Self Directed Learning in Nursing [Internet]. 2018. Available from: https://nursinganswers.net/essays/self-directed-learning-nursing-3515.php?vref=1 [Accessed: November 19, 2022]

[34] Ojekou G, Okanlawon F. Nursing students' readiness for self-directed learning and its effect on learning outcome in south-West Nigeria. Open Journal of Nursing. 2019;**9**:586-601. DOI: 10.4236/ojn.2019.96048

[35] Lee S, Kim DH, Chae SM. Self-directed learning and professional values of nursing students. Nurse Education in Practice. 2020;**42**:102647. DOI: 10.1016/j.nepr.2019.102647 Epub 2019 Oct 24

[36] Wong FMF, Tang ACY, Cheng WLS. Factors associated with self-directed learning among undergraduate nursing students: A systematic review. Nurse Education Today. 2021;**104**:104998. DOI: 10.1016/j.nedt.2021.104998 Epub 2021 Jun 5

[37] Chou FH, Chin CC. Experience of problem-based learning in nursing education at Kaohsiung Medical University. The Kaohsiung Journal of Medical Sciences. 2009;**25**(5):258-263. DOI: 10.1016/S1607-551X(09)70071-3

[38] Crawford TR. Using problem-based learning in web-based components of nurse education. Nurse Education in Practice. 2011;**11**(2):124-130. DOI: 10.1016/j.nepr.2010.10.010

[39] Choi E, Lindquist R, Song Y. Effects of problem-based learning vs. traditional lecture on Korean nursing students' critical thinking, problem-solving, and self-directed learning. Nurse Education Today. 2014;**34**(1):52-56. DOI: 10.1016/j.nedt.2013.02.012 Epub 2013 Mar 25

[40] Kokol P, Blazun H, Micetić-Turk D, Abbott PA. E-learning in nursing education—Challenges and opportunities. Studies in Health Technology and Informatics. 2006;**122**:387-390

[41] Kala S, Isaramalai SA, Pohthong A. Electronic learning and constructivism: A model for nursing education. Nurse Education Today. 2010;**30**(1):61-66. DOI: 10.1016/j.nedt.2009.06.002

[42] Kumar A, Kalal N, Rana N, Vyas H, Choudhary V, Rani R. Online learning in nursing students: Satisfaction and barriers. Journal of Education Health Promotion. 2021;**30**(10):411. DOI: 10.4103/jehp.jehp_1221_20

[43] Thapa P, Bhandari SL, Pathak S. Nursing students' attitude on the practice of e-learning: A cross-sectional survey

amid COVID-19 in Nepal. PLoS One. 2021;**16**(6):e0253651. DOI: 10.1371/journal.pone.0253651

[44] Chen B, Yang T, Wang Y, Xiao L, Changxia X, Shen Y, et al. Nursing students' attitudes toward mobile learning: An integrative review. International Journal of Nursing Sciences. 2021;**8**(4):477-485. DOI: 10.1016/j.ijnss.2021.08.004

[45] Wong AKC, Wong FKY, Chan LK, Chan N, Ganotice FA, Ho J. The effect of interprofessional team-based learning among nursing students: A quasi-experimental study. Nurse Education Today. 2017;**53**:13-18. DOI: 10.1016/j.nedt.2017.03.004 Epub 2017 Mar 9

[46] Wong E, Leslie JJ, Soon JA, et al. Measuring interprofessional competencies and attitudes among health professional students creating family planning virtual patient cases. BMC Medical Education. 2016;**16**:273. DOI: 10.1186/s12909-016-0797-8

[47] Buring SM, Bhushan A, Broeseker A, Conway S, Duncan-Hewitt W, Hansen L, et al. Interprofessional education: Definitions, student competencies, and guidelines for implementation. American Journal of Pharmaceutical Education. 2009;**73**(4):59. DOI: 10.5688/aj730459

[48] Hammick M, Freeth D, Koppel I, Reeves S, Barr H. A best evidence systematic review of interprofessional education: BEME guide no. 9. Medical Teacher. 2007;**29**(8):735-751. DOI: 10.1080/01421590701682576

[49] Mennenga HA, Smyer T. A model for easily incorporating team-based learning into nursing education. International Journal of Nursing Education Scholarship. 2010;**7**:4. DOI: 10.2202/1548-923X.1924 Epub 2010 Jan 27

[50] Roh YS, Lee SJ, Mennenga H. Factors influencing learner satisfaction with team-based learning among nursing students. Nursing & Health Sciences. 2014;**16**(4):490-497. DOI: 10.1111/nhs.12118 Epub 2014 Mar 17

[51] Cheng CY, Liou SR, Hsu TH, Pan MY, Liu HC, Chang CH. Preparing nursing students to be competent for future professional practice: Applying the team-based learning-teaching strategy. Journal of Professional Nursing. 2014;**30**(4):347-356. DOI: 10.1016/j.profnurs.2013.11.005 Epub 2013 Nov 15.

[52] Clark MC, Nguyen HT, Bray C, Levine RE. Team-based learning in an undergraduate nursing course. The Journal of Nursing Education. 2008;**47**(3):111-117. DOI: 10.3928/01484834-20080301-02

[53] Chiew-Jiat S, Fui-Ping L, Ah-Ewe L, Siew-Tiang L, Wilson T. Efficacy of team-based learning in knowledge integration and attitudes among year-one nursing students: A pre- and post-test study. Collegian. 2019;**26**(5):556-561. DOI: 10.1016/j.colegn.2019.05.003

[54] Choi KO, Park YM. The effects of team-based learning on problem solving ability, critical thinking disposition and self-directed learning in undergraduate nursing students. Journal of East-West Nursing Research. 2014;**20**(2):154-159. DOI: 10.14370/JEWNR.2014.20.2.154

[55] Qalehsari MQ, Khaghanizadeh M, Ebadi A. Lifelong learning strategies in nursing: A systematic review. Electronic Physician. 2017;**9**(10):5541-5550. DOI: 10.19082/5541

Chapter 6

The Teaching of Integrative and Complementary Practices in the Inter-Unit Modality as Curriculum Innovation

Rosemeire Sartori de Albuquerque,
Beatriz Aparecida Ozello Gutierreztwo, Eliane Ribeiro,
Christiane Borges do Nascimento Chofakian,
Renata Figueiredo de Oliveira and Giovana Araujo de Moura

Abstract

Knowing the impact of a hybrid discipline and inter-units of integrative and complementary practices for academics at the University of São Paulo. Cross-sectional quantitative research, with 62 students from USP, São Paulo, Brazil. Data collection between August and December 2021, with questionnaires via Google Form and data analysis using Excel (2016) and Likert Scale. Prevailed students aged between 22 and 25 years (38.5%), from the Obstetrics course (25.6%), with motivation (48.71%) to deepen their knowledge, adequate workload (75.0%), most interesting theme Yoga (75.0%), excellent (40.0%) evaluation strategy, and satisfied with the optional modality (65%) and inter-unit (90.0%) with recommendation of new classes (100.0%). The results showed that it was a positive experience for the students, which strengthens the implementation of the discipline in other courses.

Keywords: complementary and integrative health, educational measurement, interdisciplinary placement, integrality in health, curriculum

1. Introduction

The Integrative and Complementary Health Practices (PICS) encompass a set of health actions that aim to "encourage natural mechanisms for disease prevention, health promotion and recovery through effective and safe technologies". These practices emphasize "welcoming listening, the development of the therapeutic bond and the integration of the human being with the environment and society". Coming from different geographic, cultural, and historical origins, the PICS are based on the model of humanized care and centered on the integrality of the individual [1].

In the Brazilian scenario, from the creation of the Unified Health System (SUS) in the 1980s, the legitimization and institutionalization of PICS approaches were envisioned, while states and municipalities acquired greater autonomy in their policies and actions in health, with decentralization and popular participation. In this sense, the National Policy on Integrative and Complementary Practices (PNPIC) within the scope of the SUS was constituted based on the guidelines and recommendations of several national health conferences and also guided by the recommendations of the World Health Organization (WHO) [2].

In view of this scenario, the PICS were institutionalized in the SUS through the PNPIC, approved by Ordinance GM/MS No. 971 on May 3, 2006 (BRASIL, 2006). The policy supports a set of health practices based on the use of light technologies that encourage the person's own recovery potential. Given the cost-effectiveness, the PICS are excellent therapeutic approaches for health care in the Unified Health System, which transport other knowledge and practices into the conventional model of care, in addition to already being on the rise and increasing visibility [2].

In this way, specialist authors in the area even reinforce the innovation of the PICS to the conventional model of health, permeating that.

> *[...] "This advance can be understood as an expression of a movement that identifies itself with new ways of learning and practicing health, since these practices are characterized by interdisciplinarity and unique languages, which in general oppose each other to the highly technological vision of health that prevails in market society, dominated by health plans, whose main objective is to generate profit and fragment patient treatment into specialties that do not handle the totality of human beings in search of a remedy for their ills" (TELESI JÚNIOR, 2016, p. 99) [3].*

Parallel to this issue, humanization in health has been envisaged as a quality benchmark for comprehensive care, allowing it to overcome its technical and scientific vision and consider the individuality, dignity and rights of the health-care user.

Health, in addition to recognizing the professional as a person, establishes an individual-individual care relationship [4].

Still, it is possible to mention the importance of disciplinary plurality, which the authors point out as "the path to a broader and more global view of the human being", in relation to subjectivity in health practices and care. The PICS work precisely in the sense of contributing to disciplinary integration, with its immense variety of resources, since it "descends from an ancient tradition of continued and practically unchanged use of the same technological resources, guided by an interdisciplinary nature". This allows therefore to note the sustainability and importance of the practices [3].

However, when analyzing the scenario of Integrative and Complementary Practices in undergraduate courses in the health area in Brazil, its presence as a discipline appears to be incipient, revealing a relative lack of knowledge on the part of most professionals. For studies on the subject, according to Tesser, Sousa, and Nascimento (2018), training in PIC in Brazil is insufficient and diffuse, with limitations in supply and quality, proving to be initial and modest, far from the experience of other countries [5].

A study exemplifying this issue estimates that less than 10% of the medical courses offered in the country included PICS content in their curricula, while in the international scenario this number reached up to 80%, indicating that the teaching of PICS has been gradually introduced in courses of graduation in the area of health and, in a smaller number, in those of specialization [6].

The aforementioned perspectives, moreover, are in line with the third goal of the Healthy Development Goals, "to ensure a healthy life and the promotion of well-being for all, at all ages", by the PICS contemplating the fields of prevention, promotion, maintenance, and recovery of health, aiming at a model of humanized care centered on the integrality of the individual [7].

Similarly, teaching and training in the PICS are also in accordance with the National Curriculum Guidelines (DCNs), which provide changes in the way of teaching and learning, recommending active learning methods and the incorporation of teaching technologies, and at the same time point to the importance of critical and reflective training, committed to the institution of health policies and the needs of the population [8].

Given the above, the incipient training of Integrative and Complementary Health Practices in Brazilian universities, the congruence with the Sustainable Development Goals, and the nuances of the National Curriculum Guidelines reveal the importance of studying practices as an undergraduate discipline. Thus, emerged the present study with the objective of knowing the impact of a hybrid, innovative discipline, offered in the inter-unit mode aimed at integrative and complementary practices for academics of five courses in the area of health at the University of São Paulo.

2. Method

This is a cross-sectional quantitative study, carried out with 62 students enrolled in the undergraduate course called "Comprehensive care throughout the life cycle in the light of Integrative Practices". The discipline was elaborated, submitted, and approved in a public notice by the University of São Paulo (USP) whose proposal was to build opportunities for modern, hybrid, intra- and inter-institutional training, which would satisfy the recent demands of contemporary society in different areas of knowledge, with a view to comprehensive care, in line with the promotion of well-being for all and at all ages.

The discipline was developed in the second half of 2021 as an optional course, with a workload of 60 hours, in the hybrid format, with 16 meetings of 4 hours each for undergraduates of the Obstetrics, Gerontology, Nursing, Pharmacy, and Medicine courses at USP. It was coordinated by the campus of the São Paulo School of Arts, Sciences and Humanities at USP.

The study population consisted of all 62 enrolled students. Throughout the course, there were some dropouts, and the sample consisted of 46 participants. According to the flowchart shown in **Figure 1**.

For data collection, which took place between August and December 2021, two questionnaires were prepared and applied via Google Form. The first, carried out before the start of the first class, with the aim of characterizing the students, consisted of 12 questions covering age, profession, year of admission to the university, existence of previous contact with some of the integrative and complementary practices in health (PICS) that justified their interest in enrolling in the course, reason for taking the course, and expectations regarding classes scheduled for the semester.

The second questionnaire, applied on the last day of class, contained 26 questions, through the Google Forms platform. This had the purpose of knowing the impact of the discipline developed for the students. Questions were included regarding workload, topics and content covered, didactic strategy, evaluation methodology, and face-to-face visits and in relation to the hybrid teaching model, in addition to requesting suggestions for possible improvements and new offer of the discipline.

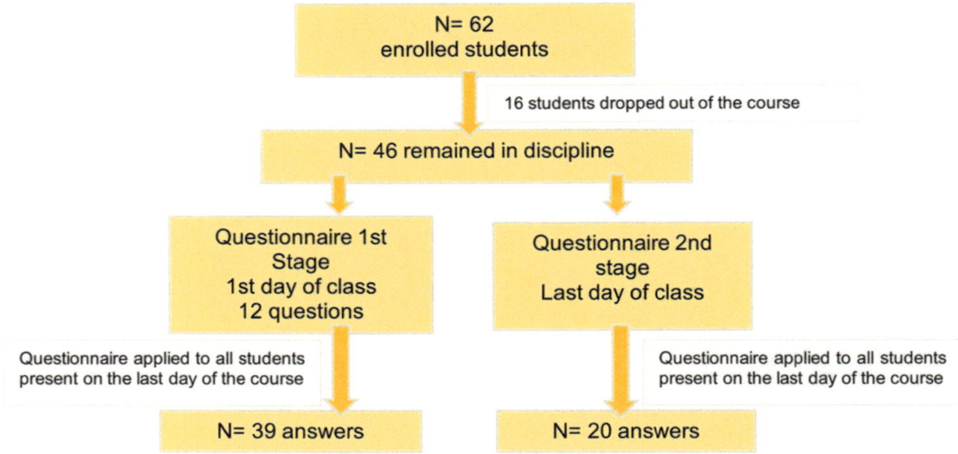

Figure 1.
Represents flow for sample size. Brazil, 2022.

In ethical terms, students were invited to participate in the present study, and data collection took place only upon acceptance and signing of the Free and Informed Commitment Term. The research was submitted and approved by the Ethics and Research Committee of the School of Arts, Sciences and Humanities of the University of São Paulo, under number 5.048.613, complying with all ethical principles required for scientific studies, including voluntary participation, privacy of participants, and confidentiality of information, in accordance with the Resolution of the National Health Council (CNS) n° 466/2012 and n° 510/2016 related to Research with Human Beings.

Dice were analyzed in Microsoft Excel 2016, using absolute numbers and proportions. The independent variables concern the student's profile (age, course, year of admission, profession, period of study, and fields of study), previous contact with integrative and complementary practices (undergraduate discipline, specialization, health services, and others), and students' perception of the discipline (workload, content covered, professors in charge, optional modality, remote teaching, inter-unit modality, topic considered the most relevant, and topic offered with better didactics). To analyze the evaluation strategy proposed in the course, a Likert scale was used, developed by the researchers, which ranged from 0 to 10, with 0 considered as poor and 10 as excellent. Finally, Word Clouds (NP) were used, which are graphic resources that simulate the frequency of terms in hypertexts, to identify what it meant for the student to have attended the discipline "Comprehensive care throughout the life cycle in the light of Integrative Practices".

3. Results

The results presented below refer to data collected from 39 students participating in the first stage of the research and 20 in the second, as represented in the **Figure 1**.

It is worth mentioning that 122 students expressed interest in the discipline; however, only 60 places could be offered, with authorization for two exchange students, totaling the number to 62 students enrolled. After presenting the evaluation strategy to be adopted, due to difficulty in completing all the tasks, 16 students dropped out, with 46 remaining until the end of the activities. The sample participating in the research consisted of the total number of students present on the first day of class and who answered the first questionnaire and the total also present on the last day of class, who answered the second questionnaire, which made up the representative sample.

The results presented in **Table 1** show that most participants were between 22 and 25 years old (38.5%), followed by 18 to 21 years old (33.3%), 30 years old or more (23.1%), and 26 to 29 years old (5 .12%).

Characterization of enrolled students	**N = 39**	
	N	**%**
Age		
18 to 21 years old	13	33.3
22 to 25 years old	15	38.5
26 to 29 years old	2	5.1
30 years or more	9	23.1
Course		
Midwifery	10	25.64
Gerontology	6	15.38
Nursing	5	12.82
Pharmacy	5	12.82
Nutrition	3	7.69
Psychology	2	5.12
Others	8	20.51
Year of joining the course		
2016	3	7.69
2017	5	12.58
2018	7	17.94
2019	11	28.2
2020	4	10.25
2021	6	15.38
Profession		
Student	25	64.1
Other professionals	14	35.9
Period of study		
1st or 2nd semester	3	15
3rd or 4th semester	1	5
5th or 6th semester	7	35
7th or 8th semester	7	35
Other semesters	2	10
Fields of study		

Characterization of enrolled students	N = 39	
	N	%
School of Arts, Science and Humanities	11	55
School of Nursing	3	15
Faculty of Public Health	3	15
Others	3	15

Table 1.
Characterization of enrolled students, according to age, course, year of admission, profession, course period, and study campus. São Paulo-SP, Brazil, 2021. (n = 39 n = 20).

Regarding the proportion of students from the different courses involved, it was observed that most (25.64%) were from the Obstetrics course, followed by Gerontology (15.38%), Nursing and Pharmacy (12.82%), Nutrition (7.69%), and Psychology (5.12%). There was also participation, to a lesser extent, by those enrolled in other USP courses, namely, Pedagogy, Dentistry, and Occupational Therapy and Speech Therapy named as others, represented together (20.51%).

As for the most prevalent year of admission to graduation, it was 2019 (28.20%), followed by 2018 (17.94%) and 2021 (15.38%). Of the participants, 64.10% were only students, and 35.89% already worked as a gerontologist, doula, researcher, floral therapist, teacher, dentist, and self-employed.

It can also be seen in **Table 1** that among the students from the different USP campuses involved, the participation (55%) of those from the School of Arts, Sciences and Humanities stood out, followed by the School of Nursing and the Faculty of Public Health and other campuses. From USP (15%), where the majority (70%) of the undergraduates was between the 5th and 8th semester of their course.

The majority (82.1%) of the students had already had previous contact with some of the program's integrative practices, where 37.7% were in health services, 31.3% with content within other undergraduate disciplines, and 15.38% in specialization, personal life, or study projects, according to the **Figure 2**.

Regarding the students' perception of the course's syllabus and content, most considered the workload and the contents covered adequate (75% and 60%, respectively) and that the professors responsible for the course were excellent (60%) and were satisfied with regard to the discipline being optional (65%) and offered inter-unit (90%), and 80% reported that there were no losses regarding the hybrid modality (**Table 2**).

The topics considered the most interesting in the students' view were Yoga (75%), followed by Acupuncture (65.0%), Floral Therapy (65.0%), and Auriculotherapy (65.0%). Also, referring to the theme offered with better didactics, Yoga was again the most cited (65.0%), followed by Aromatherapy/essential oils (60.0%), search for scientific evidence (55.0%), Map of evidence of PICs (50.0%), Traditional Chinese Medicine (50.0%), Bioenergetic (50.0%), Reflexology (50.0%), and Shantala (50.0%) (data not shown in table).

Regarding the evaluation strategy proposed in the course, most students scored 9 (40%) and 8 (20%) on the Likert Scale. In addition, the respondents unanimously agreed to recommend the subject for the next classes (100%) (data not shown in the table).

It is noteworthy that among the questions present in the questionnaire, the last one referred to the student's one-word description of the meaning for him of having the

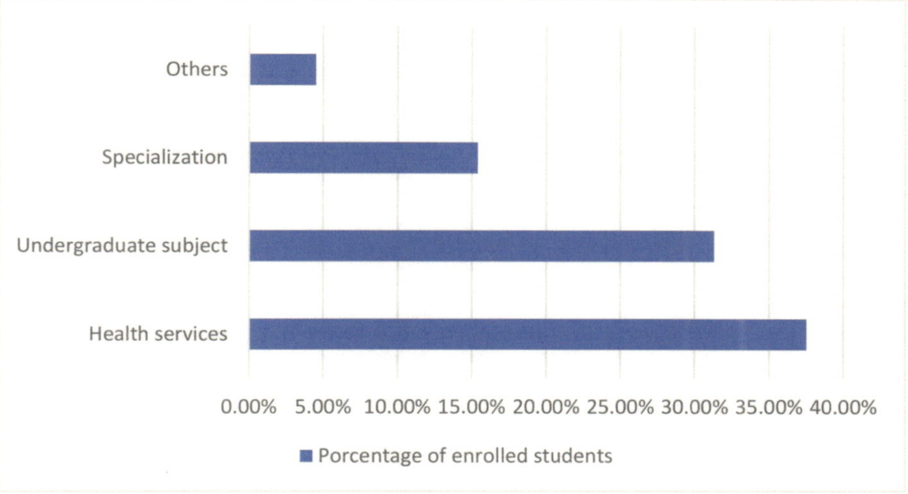

Figure 2.
Students enrolled in the course, according to previous contact with integrative and complementary health practices. São Paulo, SP, Brazil, 2021.

Enrolled students' perception	N = 39	
	N	%
Workload		
Appropriate	15	75
Good	4	20
Inadequate	1	5
Insufficient	0	0
Content covered		
Appropriate	12	60
Good	8	40
Inadequate	0	0
Insufficient	0	0
Responsible teachers		
Great	18	90
Good	2	10
Regular	0	0
Bad	0	0
Optional modality		
Satisfied	13	65
Indifferent	5	25
Dissatisfied	2	10
Teaching remote		
There were losses	16	80

Enrolled students' perception	N = 39	
	N	%
There were no damage	4	20
Inter-unit modality		
Satisfied	18	90
Indifferent	2	10
Dissatisfied	0	0

Table 2.
Students' perception of the workload, content covered, professors in charge, optional modality, remote teaching, and inter-units of the discipline "Integral Care throughout the life cycle in the light of Integrative Practices". Sao Paulo, SP, Brazil (N = 39).

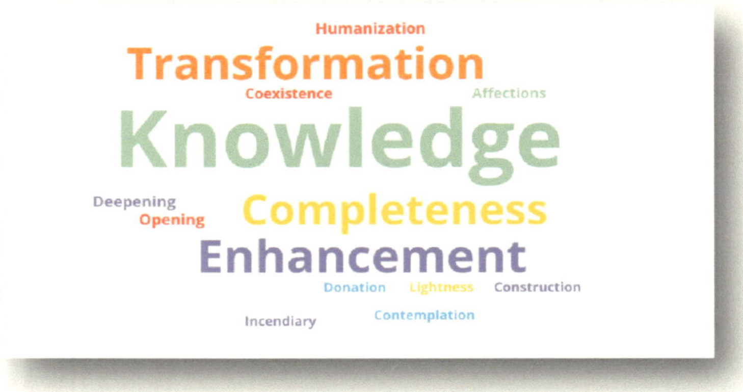

Figure 3.
Cloud of words "meaning when attending the Comprehensive Care course throughout the life cycle in the light of Integrative Practices", São Paulo -SP, Brazil, 2021.

subject studied, with "knowledge" being the most prevalent, followed by "improvement", "transformation," and "comprehensiveness" (**Figure 3**).

4. Discussion

The school environment has proven to be an opportune place for co-responsibility about the health process recognized as a social space where general information is available, in addition to allowing education for health [9].

Important initiatives corroborate the importance of developing strategies to strengthen integrative and complementary practices in health. The Project for Strengthening the National Policy on Integrative and Complementary Health Practices (PNPIC) advanced in 2022 with the perspective of designing an updated picture of the implementation of PICS in the regions of Brazil and of creating, in partnership with universities and other organizations, possibilities for training of health professionals and technical consultancy to support states and municipalities [10].

According to partial data obtained for the year 2019, PICS were offered in 17,335 services of the Health Care Network and distributed in 4297 municipalities (77%). There was an increase of 16% (2860) in the number of services compared to 2017, where 15,603 (90%) are in primary health care [11].

There are challenges in the health and health-teaching scenarios. The incorporation of integrative practices in the training of future professionals can be an important strategy to awaken, strengthen, and consolidate comprehensive care.

On the one hand, there is a growing demand for new therapeutic practices in health services, especially after 2006, with the publication of the National Policy on Integrative and Complementary Practices (PNPIC) by the Ministry of Health. The patients often seek differentiated care, beyond the conventional, but the professional is not always prepared to offer it, according to the individual needs of the population served [12].

However, the offer of PICs in undergraduate courses, in fact, has been incipient, since the number of health courses that have their teaching in their formal curriculum is reduced, and when offered, they are optional, leading to a fragility of formal education on these practices [13].

The present research showed that the proposal for the discipline integrated more courses, in addition to those of Obstetrics and Gerontology on the campus of the School of Arts, Sciences and Humanities of the University of São Paulo, with content on the different integrative and complementary practices in health, and provided an opportunity common to the different courses at USP, with a focus on promoting a more comprehensive education and with the possibility of qualification beyond the already established technical preparation. In addition, the hybrid modality offered was in line with the National Curriculum Guidelines (DCNs) that encourage changes in the way of teaching and learning, which recommend active learning methods and the incorporation of teaching technologies [8].

In this sense, the data found from the implementation of the curriculum with the insertion of the subject "Integral Care throughout the life cycle in the light of Integrative Practices" made it possible to recognize that there was an impact for enrolled students, since, when comparing the responses from the initial questionnaire applied with those from the second, it was evident that the expectations cast on the discipline were met, with emphasis on access to scientific evidence for the basis of professional practice and health care.

In view of this, the completion of the discipline provided favorable considerations to the participants, when they launched positive perspectives regarding the workload, the themes and contents addressed, teachers involved, didactics, evaluation methodology, and hybrid model offered, in addition to the face-to-face visits that took place during the course semester.

The results of the present study are in line with the findings in the literature, where they show positive points in the perception of PICs as a new field for professional performance14 Otherwise, it is also noted that.

> *[...] "the insertion of disciplines, focused on PICS, in the curricular matrices of higher education, will provide the professional with lines of work that, sometimes, become unknown, due to the direction of the courses for treatments conservative, in addition to providing them with forms of patient care in a more humane and holistic way" [14].*

According to the understanding of the undergraduates about the discipline developed, the proposal was innovative, by promoting interaction and connection between courses in the health area, by configuring inter-units, putting an end to interdisciplinarity. This perspective is discussed by authors who defend disciplinary plurality as a way to reach a broader, holistic, and global perspective of the individual. The result of this process then forms the exchange of knowledge and knowledge sharing [15].

In the same way, offering the discipline in the inter-unit mode, in addition to strengthening multidisciplinarity, could offer knowledge about the PICS made available by the Unified Health System, which are little publicized within the scope of the University of São Paulo, as well as in other public or even private institutions. In view of this, despite being advocated in the policies of the Unified Health System, as well as by the Federal Council of Nursing (COFEN), studies show a shortage of public and private institutions that offer disciplines in undergraduate courses on these practices in the state of São Paulo, location of the USP unit where the discipline involved in this research was developed [16].

For Santos and other collaborators (2022), teaching PICS at undergraduate level means contributing to the implementation of SUS principles, in addition to boosting comprehensive health care17 Thus,

> *[...] "the presentation of the PICS during graduation occurs as an awareness of the formation of individualized care, which follows bioethical principles and valuing life and which is always looking for new knowledge, but which is not limited to scientific publications, given the incipience of these to assess contexts and individualized care. Within professional experiences, learning about the importance of providing comprehensive care stands out. This offer is essential for the quality of health care, in order to break with the hospital-centered and fragmented model, in addition to re-signifying the concept of health by the users themselves. By observing the multiple field of action, the discipline manages to be useful for all health professionals, regardless of the area they choose to work in" [17].*

According to the view of some authors, the multiple field of action, regardless of the area in which the health professional works, the preparation for comprehensive care indicates adherence to a teaching that contains content that supports this care, which is mandatory in training and not as an option.

Therefore, it is known that the discipline "Integral care throughout the life cycle in the light of Integrative Practices" has met with excellence the objectives and goals proposed in its project, positively impacting the training of students, giving visibility to the University of São Paulo, and facing Integrative and Complementary Practices within the scope of the triad: teaching, research, and extension.

A limitation of the study is the fact that not all of the students responded, since only those present on the first and last day participated in the study. Therefore, the findings favor that new courses include the content of integrative practices as a subject in the curriculum so that more students take ownership of recognized and applicable practices for differentiated health care, as well as be able, as professionals, to encourage the provision of PICS as a complementary resource for the health and well-being of the population served.

5. Conclusion

The study showed that the proposal for an innovative discipline, in the interdisciplinary modality, on Integrative and Complementary Practices in Health, offered at the University of São Paulo, was considered positive for students in the health area, with a positive impact on their training. They highlighted as a positive point the workload, topics and contents addressed, teachers involved, didactics of the class taught, and evaluation strategy.

In this way, the importance of expanding content focused on the PICS to other undergraduate health courses and other institutions is verified, especially in the inter-disciplinary and mandatory nature, given the limited offer among universities, even 15 years after the institutionalization of the practices in the Unified Health in Brazil.

Acknowledgements

The development of the project and presentation of the results, which provided the presentation of this chapter, were possible with funding from the Program to Stimulate Modernization and Reformulation of Structures.

Curriculum of USP Undergraduate Courses - New Curricula for a New Time.

Notice PRG 01/2020-2021, as well as the participation of all those involved, students, teachers, monitors, and support. Our acknowledgment and thanks.

Author details

Rosemeire Sartori de Albuquerque[1*], Beatriz Aparecida Ozello Gutierreztwo[1], Eliane Ribeiro[2], Christiane Borges do Nascimento Chofakian[1], Renata Figueiredo de Oliveira[1] and Giovana Araujo de Moura[3]

1 School of Arts, Sciences and Humanities of the University of São Paulo EACH/USP, São Paulo, SP, Brazil,

2 Faculty of Pharmaceutical Sciences, University of São Paulo FCF/USP, São Paulo, SP, Brazil

3 University of São Paulo School of Nursing, EEUSP, Nurse, São Paulo, SP, Brazil

*Address all correspondence to: rosemeiresartori@usp.br

References

[1] Brazil. Ministry of Health. Historical Context of the Institutionalization of Integrative and Complementary Health Practices No Sus. National Coordination of Integrative and Complementary Health Practices (CNPICS). 2020.

[2] Brasil. Ministério da Saúde. Política nacional de práticas integrativas e complementares no SUS - PNPIC-SUS: atitude de ampliação de acesso. Brasília-DF. 2ª ed. 2015. Disponível em: http://189.28.128.100/dab/docs/portaldab/publicacoes/politica_nacional_praticas_integrativas_complementares_2ed.pdf. [Acesso em: Abril de 2022]

[3] Júnior T, Emílio. Práticas integrativas e complementares em saúde, uma nova eficácia para o SUS. Estudos avançados. 2016;**30**(86):99-112

[4] Castillo-Parra S et al. Teachers' voices seeking humanized teaching in nursing: Virtual experiences during the pandemic. Texto & Contexto-Enfermagem. 2022;**31**:1-12

[5] Tesser CD, de Sousa IMC, do Nascimento MC. Práticas integrativas e complementares na atenção primária à saúde brasileira. Saúde em debate. 2018;**42**:174-188

[6] de Azevedo E, Pelicioni MCF. Práticas integrativas e complementares de desafios para a educação. Trabalho, Educação e Saúde. 2011;**9**(3):361-378

[7] IPEA. Objetivo do Desenvolvimento Sustentável. 2019. Disponível em: https://www.ipea.gov.br/ods/ods3.html. [Acesso em: Abril de 2022]

[8] Carvalho, Amanda Cordeiro de Oliveira, et al. O planejar docente: relato sobre uso de métodos ativos no ensino de enfermagem. Rev. enferm. UFPE on line. 2016;**2016**:1332-1338

[9] Pires Laurena Moreira et al. "A enfermagem no contexto da saúde do escolar: revisão integrativa da literatura". Rev. Enferm. UERJ, Rio de Janeiro. 2012:**20**(5):668-675

[10] Brasil. Ministério da Saúde. PORTARIA N° 971, DE 03 DE MAIO DE. 2006. Disponível em: https://bvsms.saude.gov.br/bvs/saudelegis/gm/2006/prt0971_03_05_2006.html. [Acesso em: Abril de 2022]

[11] Brasil. Ministério da Saúde. Relatório de Monitoramento Nacional das Práticas Integrativas e Complementares em Saúde nos Sistemas de Informação em Saúde. 2020. Disponível em: http://189.28.128.100/dab/docs/portaldab/documentos/pics/Relatorio_Monitoramento_das_PICS_no_Brasil_julho_2020_v1_0.pdf. [Acesso em: Maio de 2022]

[12] Habimorad, Pedro Henrique Leonetti, et al. Potencialidades e fragilidades de implantação da Política Nacional de Práticas Integrativas e Complementares. Ciência & Saúde Coletiva. 2020;**25**:395-405

[13] Barboni, Viviana Graziela de Almeida Vasconcelos, and Yara Maria de Carvalho. Práticas Integrativas e Complementares em saúde na formação em Educação Física: avanços, desafios, velhos e novos embates. Saúde e Sociedade. 2021;**30**:1-6

[14] Vieira, Laís Emanuelle Bernardo, et al. "IMPLANTAÇÃO DA DISCIPLINA PRÁTICAS INTEGRATIVAS E COMPLEMENTARES EM CURSO DE GRADUAÇÃO EM FARMÁCIA." Editora Realize. 2017. p. 1-6

[15] Davila AP, Lays da Rocha Piccini. O monitor e as práticas integrativas complementares interdisciplinares. 2019

[16] Oliveira TA et al. Ensino das Práticas Integrativas e Complementares nos cursos de enfermagem do Estado de São Paulo. Nursing (São Paulo). 2020;**23**:4392-4401

[17] Santos TS et al. Ensino das práticas integrativas e complementares em saúde na enfermagem. Research, Society and Development. 2022;**11**:e311122533 6-e3111225336

Section 3

Other Trends and Developments

Chapter 7

Challenges for Nursing in Future Trends and Developments

Sandra Xavier and Lucília Nunes

Life is divided into three terms
– that which was, which is, and which will be
Let us learn from the past to profit by the present,
and from the present, to live better in the future".

– William Wordsworth

Abstract

Nurses based on a fundamental moral value which is the interest of the person—therefore, actions and interventions must take into account the needs and interests of the Other. This chapter discusses four challenges, moving from nursing epistemology to research-based practices. It is necessary to emphasize knowledge to establish a robust connection between the nurses' fields of activity. We also discuss the challenges associated with technology in learning and teaching, in telenursing or clinical nursing. The third choice we made is to enrich the development of emotional skills by sharing components and dimensions. The emotional competence was first studied in a clinical context before being extrapolated to teaching and management. To be more precise, emotional competence belongs to the subject himself as the first resource. In the fourth challenge, the environment and the world are seen from a broader perspective. We question whether improving literacy is relevant to empowering people and citizens to promote and fight for safe care and a sustainable and peaceful environment in the context of "One Health" and "One Ethics." These four trends are both challenges and horizons. Furthermore, as we approach any horizon, it gets closer until we reach a new starting point.

Keywords: nursing care, nursing research, nursing education, trends, developments

1. Introduction

Nursing, as a discipline of knowledge and liberal profession, faces, in our century, a set of challenging dimensions, with diverse origins, from the internal issues of the discipline (such as the epistemological approach, the relationship between theories and practices, the specific theoretical development of its own) to broader social issues, the social area, technology, also crossing education, management, and clinical nursing.

Without claiming to address them all, we consider it proper to propose a set of challenges, related and interconnected but also autonomous in themselves and their individual results and representations: (1) Bringing theories and practices closer together using research; (2) Technology-based teaching-learning and teleconsultation; (3) Development of emotional competencies; (4) Salutogenic perspective and environmental commitment.

1.1 Bridging theories and practices through research use

Nursing epistemology has various possibilities of approaching, and for this effect, we are focused on two relevant aspects: how we know and what we do with the produced knowledge (usually named "evidence").

We could ask anyone: people have no difficulty saying that *they know*; for example, the street where they live, the other people come across, and the places they pass through and have passed through. However, it seems that we know more than the things we had direct access to because we also think to know from the narratives of Others, from readings, and indirect learning. So, looking to improve the meaning, we can pose an apparently simple question: How do we know what we think we know? As health professionals, how do nurses know what they think they know to deliver care?

It is a kind of trigger question—"when you decide to provide care, how do you know you know?", invokes strangeness, even perplexity. Trained nurses do not usually interrogate themselves these kinds of questions. You could ask them what they base their decisions on, which would at least be more orthodox. Nevertheless, the central epistemological question is about knowledge, how we know what we think we know, and what is the validity of the knowledge we must care for people. Moreover, we realize it sounds weird.

However, "how do you know that you know?" is only a first question, and it is not despicable that when a nurse provides care, they are expected to know what they are doing, why they are doing it, and what for, as well as to be confident in the act.

Interestingly, it is often the case that nurses in postgraduate education answer this question by first saying something related to outcomes. Furthermore, when we counterargue that we cannot decide on outcomes when planning nursing care for people, they suggest other grounds: like undergraduate training, research, professional experience, the reflection of previous care experiences, imagination, intuition, and heuristic thought. In short, various sources of knowledge in Nursing [1]. Ask yourself: How do I know that I know? How did I know what I think I knew? What do I do with what I [think I] know?

There are more questions right up front: under what conditions do nurses know? How did they obtain the knowledge? How do they know it is reliable or trustworthy? When do they know, justifiably, that they know something? How do they support and justify beliefs? What are the limits of knowledge?

Saying "nursing epistemology" means we are concerned with questions regarding the nature, sources, and validity of knowledge in nursing, the study of the knowledge, and justified beliefs we hold, including questions of knowledge creation and dissemination.

Dreyfus puts it simply—"The radical gap between what is inside the mind and what is outside in the world must be mediated in order for a subject to have knowledge of the world, and epistemology is the study of this mediation" [2]. In the case of nursing, it is about considering the core of the discipline and the modes of operationalization of materialization in professional action.

As Mark Risjord put, "Nursing has two faces. To the public, nurses embody the best of modern health care. Efficient, effective, and caring nurses are at the center of the patient's experience. The other face is largely invisible to the patient, even though it has been a part of nursing since the time of Florence Nightingale. Nursing requires knowledge" [3].

Nursing education is a trajectory in which a student moves toward the construction of personal knowledge (which, let us face it, in the academic phase, tends to be more standardized than unique). The enrichment of personal knowledge comes from the personal experiences and reflective construction of the person (including knowledge about oneself) and from the study, research, and updating of knowledge. Public knowledge, as Risjord says, concerns the knowledge of a discipline that is available, having the characteristics of systematization and generalization (although these characteristics vary with the maturity of the discipline, the way it integrates new knowledge into a coherent whole and encompasses epistemological issues).

The development of nursing knowledge is oriented toward the enrichment of public knowledge since this is the foundation of the discipline. Through the development of research, nurses have long asserted ownership over the knowledge necessary for their praxis—and at this point, we must define *nursing knowledge* as the knowledge relevant to nurses, "warranted as useful and significant to nurses and patients in understanding and facilitating human health processes useful and meaningful for understanding and facilitating human responses to developmental and health processes" [4], therefore, related to the understanding, explanation, and prediction of nursing phenomena, in relation to clients and outcomes for practice.

We would agree that nursing knowledge is anchored in a multifaceted base that includes data from science (evidence and research), experience, and personal derivatives of understanding. Moreover, if it is true that scientific knowledge is acquired from research, it is not the only type of evidence that nurses use in practice (instead, in their praxis), as they also use acquired experience and their own personal learning. Therefore, describing *nursing knowledge* becomes complex because it is embedded in practice and because nursing involves a set of dynamic interactions that make us realize that we know more than we can communicate.

At this point, it makes sense to call Michael Polanyi and his concept of *tacit knowledge* is that "complete objectivity as usually attributed to the exact sciences is a delusion and is, in fact, a false ideal"[1] [5].

"We must now acknowledge belief once again as the source of all knowledge. Tacit assent and intellectual passions, the sharing of a language and cultural heritage, membership of a like-minded community: such are the impulses that shape our view of the nature of things, on which we rely for our mastery of things. No intelligence, however critical or original, can operate outside such a fiduciary framework" [6].

He then wrote *The Tacit Dimension* and was one of the first to discuss and develop the concept of tacit knowledge, identifying it as the dominant principle of all knowledge. In Latin origin, *tacitus,* from silent, expresses an implicit understanding—something that does not need to be said to be recognized. In his words, "I will reconsider human knowledge, beginning with the fact that we can know more than we can say. This fact seems obvious. But it is not easy to say exactly what it means" [7].

[1] Polanyi [5] presented a theory of knowledge, arguing three things: (a) true discovery cannot be explained by a set of rules or algorithms; (b) knowledge is not only public but also personal, in the sense that it is constructed by individuals and encompasses their emotions and passions (hence Personal Knowledge, highlighting that even in science, the intellect is linked to the contribution of personal knowledge, emotions being one of its essential components); and (c) the knowledge underlying explicit knowledge is more primary and fundamental, since all knowledge is tacit or founded on it.

For Polanyi, tacit knowledge comprises two distinct dimensions:

a. the technical, including personal skills that are commonly referred to as know-how, relates to a type of knowledge deeply rooted in action and commitment to a specific context—an art or profession, a particular technology or market, or even the activities of a work group or team; and

b. the cognitive includes mental models, emotions, values, and beliefs. These elements—which we may call cognitive structures—are embedded in us in such a way that we take them for granted, defining how we act and behave and constituting the filter through which we perceive reality. Difficult to articulate in words, the cognitive dimension of tacit knowledge shapes how we perceive the world.

Looking at us, in the discipline of Nursing, any experienced nurse can provide examples of tacit knowledge in concrete situations naturally associated with their experience.

Furthermore, we realize that tacit knowledge, which we take for granted and allows us to understand the world and discern meaning in it, can be fully utilized in clinical reasoning for at least two reasons: because it explains that a recommendation of the evidence may not be suitable for that particular person (which articulates knowledge with personalization of care) and because clinical and human experience is essential and cannot be replaced by epidemiological data and scientific literature (and we are evoking the tone of voice, the expression, the words used in the narration of the story, that each person apportions in their health-disease process and the emotions, the values, and beliefs that they also transmit when narrating the story).

Each of us knows, whatever the ways of perceiving and understanding ourselves and the world. On the one hand, knowledge concerns what is expressed, what is brought to a certain level of awareness and can be shared, communicated, and researched [8]; on the other hand, knowledge is considered a central feature of professionalism because professions are based on knowledge and disciplines are an established body of formal knowledge. Therefore, it would be essential to understand how each one develops and uses his/her professional knowledge.

In fact, it is worth calling upon Charles Taylor, who insists that knowledge is primarily the result of embodied existence and experience. The way we find ourselves in the world is cognitively shaped and contained by the fact that we are bodies, which gives us a perceptual orientation to the world from our sense organs.

In the first instance, for example, we can only see things from certain angles, although we can change the angle from which we see something by moving ourselves or the objects. Today, we know in many ways that far transcend our bodily limitations (think of the microscope, the telescope, the CAT scan, or magnetic resonance imaging). However, some are concerned that the more sophisticated forms of knowing, made possible by technologies, are incorporated into, and ultimately dependent upon, our (primitive) ontological ways of knowing.

The world around us appears as a meaningful context in which we act, interact, and pursue our purposes. Knowledge does not mean it is necessarily conscious or articulate; interpretations can be tacit and pre-reflexive. As such, they typically form the backdrop to knowledge, to be accompanied by what we might call post-reflexive knowledge. Interestingly, Charles Taylor considers that "the semantic dimension" is what allows us to express ourselves correctly, so we look for the best way to express ourselves, to say it in the right way, semantically speaking.

As for those questions regarding "How do they know they know?", "Under what conditions do they know?", "How did they obtain the knowledge?", "How do they know it is reliable or trustworthy?", "What are the limits of the knowledge?", many answers report experience, talking to colleagues and team members, validation with those they consider experts, research, and "going looking in books" as an option. That, in the first place, has appeared, above all, asking the teams' experts or clinical leaders.

Furthermore, it is relevant that once the questions have been asked, nurses begin to discuss the issue and question themselves about the knowledge they think they have and how they obtained it. In other words, they should think about *nursing epistemology*, focusing on issues related to the nature, sources, and validity of nursing knowledge, the study of the knowledge, and justified beliefs we have, including the issues of knowledge creation and dissemination.

There is a commonly used speech about the separation theory-practice or the theory-practice gap, as an expression often associated with the lack of alignment between what is available in public knowledge and what is used in individual practice [3, 9]. Moreover, we need to hold meetings to enhance and strengthen the knowledge developed through the work of researchers and the personal knowledge of nurses.

Let us clarify that the expression "theory-practice gap" has been used in at least two senses:

- In a first, more superficial sense, it is said that existing theories may be considered irrelevant to practice—and, in this sense, the theory-practice gap assumes that there is intellectual knowledge that should inform practices and that this does not happen, that the body of knowledge is not used as it should be—therefore, there is a utilization gap;

- In another sense, many nurses question the direct relevance between theoretical material and care provision, questioning the relevance, importance, or usefulness of existing research and theories—which can be referred to as the relevance gap. This relevance gap is deeper and disturbing because it affects the very foundations of the discipline and becomes an issue of nursing philosophy.

So, we need to stop saying, "there is a gap between theory and practice."

We must change our language and use other words, such as «we need to bridge between theory and practices, embedded practices with evidence and conceptual knowledge as well as research findings.

Neither practice arises independently of theory, nor does theory dispense with the realization of practice, which is not the same as saying that they must be considered the same or that they are superimposable. If the practice were the criterion of theory, it would become a sham and distort theory; if the theory were only aimed at giving pointers to practice, it would not fail to overestimate the particular, nor would it be able to resist the fascination of the casuistic.

Thus, we end up at a crossroads where the ontology of the person (complex, dynamic, inseparable from their environment, and which cannot be reduced to a health or disease situation), the ontology of nursing (due to the nature of care), and the ethical framework (due to the nature of interpersonal relationships) are interrelated.

Due to the nature of the subject who knows and the people cared for, nursing knowledge goes beyond the territory of scientific and technical knowledge, into ontology and ethics, into helping and caring relationships. However, the nursing process integrates diagnoses, interventions, and outcomes informed by scientific evidence and a wide range of therapeutic modalities. In fact, there is some space and opportunities for nurse scientists to develop.

2. Technology-based teaching-learning and telenursing

WHO defines eHealth as the "cost-effective and secure use of information and communications technologies supporting health and health-related fields, including health-care services, health surveillance, health literature, and health education, knowledge, and research. Clear evidence exists on the growing impact that eHealth has on the delivery of Health care around the world today, and how it is making health systems more efficient and more responsive to people's needs and expectations" [10].

Before the COVID-19 pandemic, it was assumed that the convergence between technology and health care brings indisputable benefits, namely faster and easier access to care and health information, greater control of the user over his health information as well as in greater efficiency in the provision of care and the development of clinical and scientific research.

"The unprecedented spread of mobile technologies, as well as advancements in their innovative application to address health priorities, has evolved into a new field of *eHealth*, known as *mHealth*. According to the International Telecommunication Union, there are now close to 5 billion mobile phone subscriptions in the world, with over 85% of the world's population now covered by a commercial wireless signal" [11].

We are surrounded by smart technology (and smart means "Self-Monitoring Analysis and Reporting Technology"). The use of information and communication technologies (ICT) in health and health-related fields aims to enhance the quality, efficiency, and effectiveness of health-service management. Referring eHealth technology could be presented as a set of overlapping groups [12], including assistive technologies, safety and social technologies, Health technologies, Self-activation and personal development technologies, Design-for-all and ambient assisted living (AAL) technologies, Gerontechnology, Hospital technology, and EHR systems.

Inevitably, if the social and health reality has changed with the increasing use of technology, education cannot remain indifferent to or on the fringes of these developments.

The pandemic context and our learnings during the lockdown and social isolation show us the multiple uses of technologies to bring people closer and to teach and learn, to provide and to access clinical care or support in crisis (or just because they feel to need).

Also, the delivery of health care and nursing care, especially when distance is a critical factor, becomes easier to connect digitally. Some things we learn during the pandemic, such as the *time economy* of online meetings, could become part of our day-by-day.

Technology usage in teaching and learning has risen to its peak recently, given the current coronavirus disease 2019 pandemic and its social distancing protocols. Higher education institutions, including nursing education institutions globally, have resorted to online learning to continue teaching and learning amidst the COVID-19 pandemic.

However, we need to distinguish between "emergency remote learning" during the pandemic and distance learning, considering that synchronous digital media functions as face-to-face. Being in a synchronous online class and teaching at a distance is different.

Portable digital assistants and technology usage have become an integral part of contemporary teaching and learning—cloud computing, which includes YouTube, Google Apps, Dropbox, and Twitter, has become the reality of today's teaching and learning and has noticeably improved higher education, including nursing education [13].

Several studies have highlighted the benefits of technology usage in nursing education associated with its exponential growth; technology use in teaching and learning is flexible, minimizes traveling, and thus is cost-effective [14].

However, a gap in informatics expertise among nursing students, practicing staff, and faculty has been noted globally, which reduces the potential for nurses to utilize technology to enhance patient care and digital health was identified as an area that needs investment. We need to find ways to incorporate digital health into a pedagogic framework grounded in the spiral learning approach [15].

Furthermore, all of us, nursing teachers, are aware of technology usage in clinical settings, which can facilitate work-integrated learning and access to recent studies and guidelines (for example, for allowing access to journals and databases).

Nevertheless, nurse managers and educators feel that technology usage in nursing education is disruptive, mainly when used in clinical settings. However, we need to distinguish it from non-proficiency regarding its use, which could be a huge factor influencing its counterproductivity [16].

With the conscience that, in a very high probability, nursing students have a smartphone in their pockets, and teachers could also think of most clients or patients with smartphones. Some of them will use it to contact their family nurse or the nurse that is a reference for them to manage their individual care plan. So, it will become a challenge to use technology for health and nursing care purposes, reviewing our legal and ethical frameworks to include technology. Because we live through a digital transition, neither nursing education nor practice will remain on the side-line or immune to this considerable transformation.

3. Emotional competencies development

Our first incursions into the area of emotional competence were related to an investigation in which we focused on the nurses' professional performance and the contexts that are experienced to make it possible to mean the nurses' emotional competence in palliative care units [17].

Understanding emotions as figures of human behavior is one of the major objectives for those who develop their professional activity with and for people. Emotions constitute a permanent challenge to the human being's ability to think about himself/herself and his/her relationship with the world. Emotion only increased as a field of research in Nursing after the 90s of the last century.

Nowadays, many authors consider the integration and development of emotions essential in various areas of life, from training contexts to care contexts. Initially, the major focus of Nursing studies was on emotional strategies to enhance the provision of comfort care, patient information, and empowerment, as well as on identifying nurses' and patients' emotional experiences, thus leaving room for the nurses' emotional competence.

Emotions are not rational acts, so they are not (direct) causes of cognition. They generate feelings and rational acts, which are used for learning, that is, they are initiators of the process (of learning). As an organism faces specific challenges and opportunities, emotions immediately respond. The feeling related to them provides this as a mental alert. Feelings amplify the impact of a given situation, enhance learning, and increase the likelihood that similar situations can be anticipated [4]. In this sense, associating the emotional mind with the rational mind guides us toward the emotional matrixes as the rudder of human behavior and professional performance.

Learning and emotional development assume themselves as an important vector in the life of the human being, helping to experience daily life with emphasis on intellectual capacity and the establishment of significant interpersonal relationships.

However, emotions do not depend only on the type of circumstances in which the human being lives but instead on the evaluation of these circumstances involving a substantial modification. They occur when the person perceives very significant changes in the context that he experiences. From this function, it becomes possible to inscribe emotions in the sphere of the regulatory functions of behavior and personal and professional performance.

In this study [17], we identified and further developed a set of skills that allow knowing, regulating, achieving, and managing emotional phenomena to build and maintain interpersonal relationships in an emotional environment, which conceptualize the nurses' emotional competence. Let us consider the findings of those five dimensions:

1. emotional knowledge, recognized as the ability to know personal and Other's emotions and what their impact is on the emotion-cognition-behavior triad, identifying the following units of competence associated with it: (1) Identifies and locates personal emotions; (2) Identifies and locates emotions of Others, and (3) Identifies behaviors that generate emotions;

2. emotional regulation, the capacity to regulate emotional expressiveness to generate positive emotions, identifying the following competence units associated with it: (1) Expresses emotions; (2) Regulates manifestation; (3) Manages emotional conflicts, and (4) Self-generates positive emotions;

3. "emotional autonomy" is assumed as the capacity to attain emotional autonomy, to build day-to-day life with positive emotional tones, identifying the following competence units associated with it: (1) Builds positive day-to-day life; (2) Acts with emotional involvement; (3) Faces obstacles; (4) Builds emotional relations, and (5) Reflects in the face of the context;

4. "Social competence" is assumed as the ability to build and maintain interpersonal relationships, accepting individual choices. The description of the emotional dimension allows us to identify the following competence units associated with it: (1) Adopts listening attitudes; (2) Initiates and maintains communication; (3) Accepts choices; (4) Maintains emotional sharing, and (5) Regulates the experience;

5. "Life skills and well-being" is assumed as the capacity to manage personal defense mechanisms, organizing thoughts and attitudes to achieve balance and well-being. The description of the emotional dimension allows identifying the following units of competencies associated with it: (1) Defines Goals; (2) Takes decisions; (3) Identifies needs and resources; and (4) Promotes significant activities.

The emotional phenomena experienced are (important) circumstances that should guide human behavior. Emotional experiences are essential to access the meaning and sense we attribute to experiences. Therefore, the symbiotic relationship between knowledge, reflection, and valuation attributes meaning and power (strength) to the interpersonal relationships built.

The experience of tension and suffering requires nurses to know how to manage the associated emotional states to adapt their behavior and, consequently, the self-control required for the desired emotional regulation given the experience. However, it is essential to recognize the internal resources that allow (and facilitate) emotional regulation, to develop the ability to reflect on the various emotional shades experienced in this context of professional activity and, consequently, achieve emotional (self)regulation under the experience, focusing on generating positive emotions.

A few years later, we wrote a paper "Meaning assigned to Emotional Competence of the Nurse: an empirical study and impact on education" [18]. Emotional education is a permanent educational process, which should start in the family, then go through academic education and, consequently, professional life, which is influenced by the evolution of society (which naturally includes the family, the groups, and the school).

The challenge of emotional education is for the person to feel and recognize that the genesis of emotional development is centered on looking at oneself, assuming the understanding of what happens inside as a major objective. This means that it enhances the encounter with oneself and provides relationships with the surrounding contexts—school, family, and/or professional, and/or professional contexts.

Thus, the search for an integral human being stimulates the discovery of a balance between emotion and reason through emotional education in intrinsic connection with academic education. Therefore, it is considered fundamental to promote the need to explore and enhance the balance between people's cognitive rationale and emotions (students and/or professionals) in schools, families, and organizations.

By promoting emotional and intellectual growth, emotional education promotes the reflexive control of emotions. Personal competence is not only a competence of the emotions but also a competence of the mind—and emotional competence results from the permanent educational process that provides the knowledge (emotional knowledge) to recognize the importance of moderating negative (unpleasant) emotions and valuing positive (pleasant) emotions without repressing them in any case.

For example, the current reality in undergraduate curricula shows that the syllabus is filled with numerous (all relevant) themes, accompanied by a lack of understanding of the subject "emotional competence". The same is true for postgraduate study syllabus unless the subject is directly related to it.

Emotions could influence nursing decision-making and action, and nurses' emotional ability affects every nursing intervention. Also, it might impact the learning quality, ethical decision-making and critical thinking of nursing students, evidence and knowledge use in practice, the quality of patient care, and patient outcomes [19]. Besides palliative care, which we have already focused on, also other clinical contexts, such as in critical situations, are examples of the need to integrate emotional competence into training programs [20]. Some studies evidenced the relevance of emotional competence in the clinical ability in internships [21] as newly graduated nurses [22].

Nurses' emotional competence skills affect personal satisfaction, autonomy, interpersonal relationship skills, self-control, problem-solving, and positive mental health elements. They found solutions to problems easily by developing positive interpersonal relationships, utilizing effective coping skills, and were less affected by adverse situations. Nurses with emotional competence skills include making conscious decisions and developing and maintaining a care strategy.

Numerous studies stated a significant relationship between emotional competence skills and pro-social behaviors—which means the person acts for the benefit of others and is conducive to social harmonies, such as helping, cooperating, sharing, and comforting. Moreover, this could positively promote the mental health of those who engage in it and those who receive it, as well as the development of human society [23]. Nursing leaders must be emotionally competent in order to encourage and foster innovative behavior among their staff. In order to increase productivity and efficiency, leaders must motivate and inspire their employees [24]. The nurses' training and emotional education are assumed to optimize the quality of care provided by these professionals, so it is reiterated that the curriculum should focus on a paradigm of emotional education as cross-cutting themes for different areas of knowledge.

Emotional learning supports nurses in making decisions in their life (personal and professional), and the reference to subjective well-being as a positive consequence of emotional development is unanimous. With this purpose, emotional education allows nurses to (reflexively) control their emotions to promote their emotional and intellectual growth, being the matrix for increasing their level of emotional competence. The complexity and demand of care contexts require increasingly differentiated professionals, and the organizational dynamics should enable the growth of the professionals and, consequently, the development of organizational competencies.

4. Salutogenic perspective and environmental commitment

We hesitate in the designation of this challenge. This could be health literacy, which refers, broadly, to the ability of individuals to "gain access to, understand, and use information in ways which promote and maintain good health" [25] for themselves, their families, and their communities. As a result, health literacy is more than a resource for individuals.

Healthy behaviors and information about services and information are more likely to be adopted by people with higher health literacy levels. As a result, health literacy empowers individuals to protect themselves, their families, and their communities.

Improving health literacy in populations enables citizens to take an active role in improving their health, engage in community action for health, and push governments to address health and health equity issues. The Sustainable Development Goals do not include a specific target for health literacy. Efforts to raise health literacy will be critical in realizing the 2030 Agenda fully. In other words, health literacy is a valuable tool that empowers individuals and communities to improve their health status and achieve sustainable development.

Empowering citizens in health literacy is not about diseases and sickness—we need a salutogenic perspective focused on health promotion and prevention.

Literacy, which can be defined as the ability to use the skills taught and learned, is a determinant of individual and collective behaviors and participation in society. When applied to health, literacy enhances the capacity to make the necessary decisions for autonomous health management [26]. Health literacy can also be extended to communities while considering social and cultural contexts. Here, the concept of critical health literacy emerges. This concept considers the overall picture and thus enables people to make decisions about their individual health and the health of their community [27]. Due to the widespread use of technologies, health literacy should also emphasize digital tools as a way to promote health-related decision-making.

Research and evaluation of strategies and characteristics of interventions that use new information technologies to personalize information and promote behavior change are urgently needed. Health promotion, risk reduction, chronic disease control, and improper access to emergency services are all areas where these interventions can make a direct impact [28].

A challenge arises for national health systems—to adopt an approach centered on different contexts (personal and community) of health promotion and surveillance, leveraging technology to facilitate fruitful, effective, and motivational interventions, and providing interactive digital repositories for health promotion and e-consultations, for instance.

The Ottawa Charter for Health Promotion was adopted in 1986 to enable people to improve their health and well-being by creating healthier and more sustainable environments for living, working, studying, and playing. The slogan: "Health for All and All for Health" to achieve this transformative Agenda 2030, all actors need to be engaged in a new global partnership that leaves no one behind.

The environment is a key concept (meta-paradigmatic) in Nursing. The environment is an umbrella concept made up of human, physical, political, economic, cultural, and organizational elements, which condition and influence lifestyles and impact the concept of health.

Nurses focus their intervention on the complex interdependence of person/environment and in delivering safe care.

5. Conclusion

We considered four key challenges;

- Bridging theories and practices using research

The focus and relevance of Nursing epistemology, the construction of personal knowledge in education and experience practices, ending the speech about "gaps" between theory and practices and prefer the idea of bridging between theories and practices mediated by research findings. Due to the nature of the subject who knows and the people cared for, nursing knowledge goes beyond the territory of scientific and technical knowledge, into ontology and ethics, into helping and caring relationships. The nursing process integrates diagnoses, interventions, and outcomes informed by scientific evidence and a wide range of therapeutic modalities. In fact, there is some space and opportunities for nurse scientists to develop.

- Technology-based teaching-learning and teleconsultation

Technology usage in teaching and learning has risen to its peak recently, given the current coronavirus disease 2019 pandemic and its social distancing protocols. Higher education institutions, including nursing education institutions globally, have resorted to online learning to continue teaching and learning. So, it will become a challenge to use technology for health and nursing care purposes, reviewing our legal and ethical frameworks to include technology. Because we live through a digital transition, neither nursing education nor practice will remain on the side-line or immune to this considerable transformation.

- Emotional skills development

Nurses' emotional competence skills affect personal satisfaction, autonomy, interpersonal relationship skills, self-control, problem-solving, and positive mental health elements. They found solutions to problems easily by developing positive interpersonal relationships, utilizing effective coping skills, and were less affected by adverse situations. Nurses with emotional competence skills include making conscious decisions and developing and maintaining a care strategy.

- Salutogenic perspective and environmental engagement

We need a salutogenic perspective focused on health promotion and prevention. The slogan: "Health for All and All for Health" to achieve this transformative Agenda 2030, all actors need to be engaged in a new global partnership that leaves no one behind. The environment is a key-concept umbrella made up of human, physical, political, economic, cultural, and organizational elements, which condition and influence lifestyles and impact the concept of health. Developing health literacy, particularly concerning the profitability of technology, is one of the most significant challenges facing national health systems today as a way of empowering individuals and communities to improve their health status.

Ethical issues will have to be considered in its implementation and development, as well as the protection and safeguard of human rights.

Author details

Sandra Xavier[1]* and Lucília Nunes[2,3]

1 Escola Superior de Enfermagem de Lisboa/CIDNUR – Nursing Research, Innovation and Development Center of Lisbon, Portugal

2 School of Health, Polytechnic Institute of Setúbal, Nursing Department, Setúbal, Portugal

3 NURSE'IN – UIESI Nursing Research Unit for South and Islands, Setúbal, Portugal

*Address all correspondence to: sandraxav@sapo.pt

References

[1] Nunes L. Para uma epistemologia de Enfermagem. 2nd ed. Lusociência & SaBooks; 2020

[2] Dreyfus H. Taylor's (Anti-) epistemology. In: Abbey R, editor. Charles Taylor. Cambridge University Press; 2004. p. 52

[3] Risjord M. Nursing Knowledge. Science, Practice, and Philosophy. Wiley-Blackwell; 2010. p. 2

[4] Reed P, Lawrence L. Nursing Knowledge and Theory Innovation: Advancing the Science of Practice. Springer Publishing Company. 2008. p. 423

[5] Polanyi M. Personal Knowledge: Towards a Post-Critical Philosophy. London: Routledge & Kegan; 1958. p. 28

[6] Polanyi M. Personal knowledge. University of Chicago Press; 1958. pp. 280-281. We must now recognize belief once more as the source of all knowledge. Tacit assent and intellectual passions, the sharing of an idiom and of a cultural heritage, affiliation to a like-minded community: Such are the impulses which shape our vision of the nature of things on which we rely for our mastery of things. No intelligence, however critical or original, can operate outside such a fiduciary framework

[7] Polanyi M. The Tacit Dimension. London: Routledge & Kegan Paul; (1966/1997, p. 136). 1966. I shall reconsider human knowledge by starting from the fact that we can know more than we can tell. This fact seems obvious enough; but it is not easy to say exactly what it means

[8] Chin K. Knowledge Is a Representation of Knowing That Is Collective Judged by Standards and Criteria Shared. 2011. p. 251

[9] Kim HS. Putting theory into practice: Problems and prospects. Journal of Advanced Nursing. 1993;**18**:1632-1639

[10] World Health Organization: Strategy 2004-2007-eHealth for health-care delivery. World Health Organization (WHO). Available from: http://www.asksource.info/resources/ehealth-health-care-delivery-strategy-2004-2007

[11] WHO. mHealth. New horizons for health through mobile technologies. 2011. Available from: https://www.who.int/goe/publications/goe_mhealth_web.pdf

[12] Nunes L, Cerqueira A, Franco H. A complete guide to assistive Technology for the Elderly – At least, by now. In: García-Alonso J, Fonseca C, editors. Gerontechnology IV. Contributions to the Fourth International Workshop on Gerontechnology, IWoG 2021. Springer; 2022. pp. 190-202

[13] Hashim H. Application of technology in the digital era education. International Journal of Research in Counseling and Education. 2018;**2**(1):1-5. DOI: 10.24036/002za0002

[14] Gause G, Mokgaola IO, Rakhudu MA. Technology usage for teaching and learning in nursing education: An integrative review. Curationis. 2022;**45**(1):a2261. DOI: 10.4102/curationis.v45i1.2261

[15] O'Connor S, LaRue E. Integrating informatics into undergraduate nursing education: A case study using a spiral learning approach. Nurse Education in Practice. 2021;**50**:102934. DOI: 10.1016/j.nepr.2020.102934

[16] Forehand JW, Miller B, Carter H. Integrating mobile devices into the nursing classroom. Teaching and Learning in Nursing. 2017;**12**(1):50-52. DOI: 10.1016/j.teln.2016.09.008

[17] Xavier S, Nunes L, Basto ML. Emotional competence of the nurse: The significance of the construct. Pensar Enfermagem. 2014;**18**(2):3-19

[18] Xavier S, Nunes L. Meaning assigned to emotional competence of the nurse: Empirical study and impact on education. Revista Ibero-Americana de Saúde e Envelhecimento. 2016;**2**(2):620-636

[19] Kozlowski D, Hutchinson M, Hurley J, Rowley J, Sutherland J. The role of emotion in clinical decision making: An integrative literature review. BMC Medical Education. 2017;**17**(1):255. DOI: 10.1186/s12909-017-1089-7

[20] Soeima S. Capacidades de competência emocional dos enfermeiros no cuidar da pessoa em situação crítica (Nurses' emotional skills when providing medical care for people in a critical condition). Dissertação Mestrado Enfermagem Pessoa em Situação Crítica. 2021. Available from: https://hdl.handle.net/1822/76209

[21] Dou S, Han C, Li C, Liu X, Gan W. Influence of emotional intelligence on the clinical ability of nursing interns: A structural equation model. BMC Nursing. 2022;**21**(1):149. DOI: 10.1186/s12912-022-00933-y

[22] Kukkonen P, Leino-Kilpi H, Koskinen S, Salminen L, Strandell-Laine C. Nurse managers' perceptions of the ability of newly graduated nurses: A scoping review. Journal of Nursing Management. 2020;**28**(1):4-16. DOI: 10.1111/jonm.12891

[23] Wang H, Wu S, Wang W, Wei C. Emotional intelligence and prosocial behavior in college students: A moderated mediation analysis. Frontiers in Psychology. 2021;**12**:713227. DOI: 10.3389/fpsyg.2021.713227

[24] Carragher J, Gormley K. Leadership and emotional intelligence in nursing and midwifery education and practice: A discussion paper. Journal of Advanced Nursing. 2016;**73**(1):85-96

[25] Nutbeam D. Health promotion glossary. Health Promotion International. 1998;**13**(4):349-364. DOI: 10.1093/heapro/13.4.349 cf. Health Promotion Glossary. Available from: https://www.who.int/publications/i/item/WHO-HPR-HEP-98.1

[26] Sykes S, Wills J, Rowlands G, Popple K. Understanding critical health literacy: A concept analysis. BMC Public Health. 2013;**13**:150

[27] Chinn D. Critical health literacy: A review and critical analysis. Social Science & Medicine. 2011;**73**(1):60-67. Available from: https://pubmed.ncbi.nlm.nih.gov/21640456/

[28] Costa A et al. A strategy for the promotion of health literacy in Portugal centered around the life-course approach: The importance of digital tools. Portuguese Journal of Public Health. 2019;**37**(1):50-54. Available from: https://www.karger.com/Article/Pdf/500247

Chapter 8

Modern Times in Point of Care Diagnostics

Wolter Paans

Abstract

This chapter describes the growing influence of point-of-care diagnostics (POCD) on the daily lives of citizens, their immediate families, and healthcare providers. With a view to the future, the most important contemporary developments in this field are discussed, such as noninvasive sensor technology in the diagnostic process, practical examples of point-of-care diagnostics (POCD), including the quantify-self movement and infrared technology. Cost-effectiveness, adoption of POCD, and the contribution of POCD innovations to self-management and health literacy are also discussed. Developments in which deep learning and artificial intelligence are used to make the diagnostic results more reliable are also conferred, such as the development of point-of-care Internet diagnostics. The discussion of professional advice dilemma's in POCD, the patient's appreciation of POCD, and ethical and philosophical considerations conclude this chapter.

Keywords: point-of-care diagnostics, bedside testing, quantify-self, diagnostic technology, self-management, infrared diagnostics, Internet diagnostics, adoption

1. Introduction

The gradually more aging population, as well as the demand for self-management, calls for new and creative possibilities to better monitor health processes in a preventive way and to better monitor recovery processes after a period of illness. Technology-driven diagnostics are becoming increasingly important through making informed decisions regarding the treatment of patients [1, 2]. This chapter describes the development of technological diagnostic support in general and examines more precisely its significance for the patient, his immediate family, and the healthcare professional.

Much of the technological support for diagnostics can be summarized under "point-of-care diagnostics" (POCD) [3, 4]. This is, therefore, the focus of this chapter.

In this chapter, the concept of "POCD" is interpreted broadly. This concerns developments in which technology is used for rapid, noninvasive diagnostics where the result is immediately available for the patient and his immediate family and/or the healthcare professional. When a central laboratory analyzes a test, there is generally a lead time between administering the test and receiving the test results at the end user of the test (i.e. a healthcare professional or patient). In the case of POCD, the end user receives the test results immediately, without significant delay.

The use of POCD can increasingly be seen as an important part of regular diagnostics, although it is not yet widely implemented in education curricula or in the (nursing) care process. This chapter can be regarded as an introduction to a modern view of POCD.

The following topics will be discussed in turn:

- Point-of-care testing (POCT) as part of POCD
- Essence of technology in the diagnostic process
- Practical examples of POCD
- POCD and cost-effectiveness
- Adoption of POCD
- What should a POCD innovation contribute to?
- Point-of-care Internet diagnostics
- Professional advice dilemma in POCD
- The patient's appreciation of POCD

2. POCT as part of POCD

In the literature, a difference is noted between point-of-care testing (POCT) and point-of-care diagnostics (POCD). At POCT, the focus is on the measurement and the (use of the) measuring instrument and received data. In addition, it is often related to the replacement of laboratory test testing to bedside testing. "POCD" is a broader concept. It is about the entire diagnostic process in which technology at hand has a supporting role. You could say that "point-of-care diagnostics" is the entire (academic) field of knowledge that focuses on technological support where directly aggregated diagnostic results are delivered in a way that is directly and relatively easy to interpret in the context of the subject. This field of knowledge also includes the way in which such diagnostic test results can be used to achieve self-management, self-reliance, a better physical and mental condition, and more resilience or less vulnerability. It can also contribute to a higher level of health literacy and better family support.

So, point-of-care testing (POCT) is the test-related technology used in POCD (POCT, also "rapid bedside testing" or "rapid test"). The actions are performed outside specific test centers by, for example, nurses and regularly not by laboratory personnel.

Today, POCT is no longer just about tests based on, for example, a venipuncture, finger prick, or urine sample. It can also involve diagnostic tests that are performed on the basis of biosensors, thermal measurements, and Internet-related information exchange. Still, the most well-known "rapid bedside tests" are measuring body temperature, blood pressure, and blood gas saturation and measuring glucose in blood and urine [1–4].

3. Essence of technology in the diagnostic process

The ability to accurately determine the nature (cause and consequence) of a health problem in order to plan, implement, and evaluate appropriate treatment and care provision has been regarded as one of the most essential basic professional competences in the field of health professionals in the medical, paramedical, allied healthcare, and nursing domains.

However, recent research has shown that diagnostic skills and applications can regularly be improved in practice, which means that optimally appropriate care is not always available. Preconditions for appropriate care are, in particular, diagnostic (reasoning) skills based on declarative, procedural, and metacognitive knowledge that is made operational and is visibly expressed in a care process.

The application of technology within the diagnostic process is steadily increasing. However, this development is still often viewed separately from the empirical, symptomatic diagnostics, such as abductive diagnostics, in which a diagnosis is made mainly on the basis of intuitive, inductive, deductive, and cognitive methods.

The wish is to continue the abovementioned critical reasoning but, if possible, to expand it synergistically in the areas of knowledge as follows:

1. The use of POCD to better involve patients as well as family members in the diagnosis. So, more *Social Diagnostics* with the aim of providing appropriate care for vulnerable recipients and their relatives, addressing the values and wishes of the patient's as well as the relatives. Involving family members in all kinds of conditional measurements of the patient concerned, for instance, can have a stimulating and motivating effect on undertaking (revalidation) activities. The use of an additional genogram application (smartphone app) providing information about the family structure, and who might be able to support the patient during revalidation activities, can provide insight in the care needed in this regard for everyone involved, professionals as well as family members. Further on, to involve patients more specifically in the possibility of performing self-measurements, by giving them specific explanations and advice regarding the positive consequences of achieved results, so that better understanding can be developed in (preventive) health behavior.

2. The use of POCD to support *professional diagnostics* to be accurately and timely informed about the patient's health status. This can be of great importance in various sectors. Think of the simple blood glucose and saturation checks that ambulance personnel perform, for the remote monitoring of chronically ill single patients by nurse specialists and general practitioners (GPs). Health professionals can use the principles of POCD to tailor the care planning more related to the personal health context of patients and their relatives.

3. The use of POCD as a part of *diagnostic technology* where, for example, tiny robots can have an additional detecting function. For example, in a hemiplegic patient, the awareness that the bladder is almost full can be announced in a friendly, personal spoken way. Then, a self-catheterization can be considered at the right time (not too early or too late or too often) before going shopping. So, the aim is to use diagnostic technology in the (health)care and treatment plan appropriately, whereby the technological application is not an end in itself,

but where goals are formulated that are holistic in nature, patient-oriented, and that demonstrably support patient empowerment, self-management, improved health literacy throughout the entire healthcare chain, and further life cycle.

4. Practical examples of POCD

There are many possibilities in the field of POCD. Very well-known are of course the virus testers, the pregnancy tests, and the aforementioned blood glucose tests. However, there are interpretations of how POCD could also be understood that are related to existing adjacent knowledge areas such as the "quantify-self movement."

4.1 Quantify-self movement

In addition, the "quantify-self movement" can be mentioned; the use of the so-called activity trackers (ATs). Activity trackers (ATs) can play an essential role in supporting patients in self-management. ATs can, for instance, contribute in dealing with the nursing diagnosis of "sedentary lifestyle" in patients with heart failure or diabetes.

ATs are small, noninvasive devices that are mostly worn on the wrist. The number of steps users take along with other health measures is registered as a variable related to physical activity. Mostly in combination with an associated mobile application, this gives the person in question insight into their own health behavior.

ATs may be a promising addition to the care process enhancing the physical activity patterns of patients. Using ATs, nurses can use a tool to deliver tailored treatment to patients enhancing their capacity for self-management [5].

4.2 How to implement point-of-care diagnostics: A quantify-self (QS) example

There are various frames of reference on the basis of which the relationship can be established between the use of POCD and its individual application in the care plan. In the following overview (see **Table 1**), which is an extraction from a table previously published in the *International Journal of Nursing and Health Care Research* (vol. 5, p. 1312), a classification system for nurses has been used as reference. This concerns the following nursing classification: NANDA-I for diagnoses; Nursing Intervention Classification (NIC) for interventions; and Nursing Outcome classification (NOC) for nursing outcomes.

In the context of this chapter, the use of ATs can be seen as part of POCD; the point here is not only to look at the (benefits of the) measurement itself, but also to ensure careful implementation in the personal care plan. It is just an example; in many technological diagnostic applications, it can be related in such a way to a knowledge framework and a process-based use.

This approach could potentially catalyze the adoption and implementation of healthcare technology support in general. The propensity to use a technological tool is greater if a direct relationship with the benefits for the end users can be established (**Figure 1**).

4.3 Infrared

There are also POCD developments in the field of infrared measurements. The forehead thermometer is an example of this, although some questions can still be asked about the specificity of the measurements [6].

Assessment Physical Activity (PA) • Insufficient interest in PA. • Insufficient knowledge of benefits of PA. • Insufficient motivation. • Insufficient resources for PA. • Insufficient training for PA.	*Functions of Activity Trackers (AT) related to Assessment* • Objective registration of PA (steps/day), heart frequency, sedentary time, active time. • Awareness in PA and active/sedentary time for the client and health professional.
Diagnosis PA Physical activity level is lower than recommended: Sedentary lifestyle at less than 300 steps/day. • Physical deconditioning. • Preference for activity in low level.	*Functions of AT related to Diagnosis* • Can be used to assess a sedentary lifestyle based on steps/day and sedentary time. • Identify client groups at risk. • Begin preventive actions to enhance awareness and level of PA.
Interventions PA Explain the effect of PA on body functioning and well-being to the client. • Determine the possible barriers to being physically active. • Begin an activity with a warm up and end with a cool down. • Check vital signs such as heart rate before starting exercise. • Assist the client from the beginning to the last part of the exercise. • Recommend keeping a record of activity. • Suggest that the client have an exercise Buddy. • Encourage involvement in active forms of social activities.	*Functions of AT related to Interventions* • Feedback function to client. • Continue monitoring of goals. • Enhances self-management and self-esteem. • Possible positive effect on behavior change. • Sharing data with health professional and other AT users to support.
Outcomes PA • Increase awareness or knowledge on • importance and benefits of PA. • Identify self-monitoring techniques. • Engagement in planned exercise programs. • Increase gradually in PA. • Improve PA, mental, social, and emotional • functioning of the body.	*Functions of AT related to Outcomes* • Define SMART outcomes based on the • individual client, their needs using the AT. • AT stimulates the client to meet their goal, and enhances motivation. • AT provides reminders to meet the individual goals.

Table 1.
Activity trackers as part of POCD in the personal care plan [5].

Superficial inflammation can now also be detected with infrared applications. This is being developed, for example, for the better detection of wound healing in burn patients. In this regard, nurses have recently been able to use the so-called hyperspectral imaging (HSI) cameras. Recordings from such a camera, which was developed by NASA, can provide insight into where wound exudate accumulates. The blood flow and oxygen supply in and around the wound area can also be provided relatively easily, without being burdensome for the patient [7].

The blood circulation measurement in the foot in diabetic patients is also an example of POCD. It was already known in the first century BC that local temperature

> *"Now that I can see how many miles I walk on foot, I'm in a kind of competition with myself; I experience too few steps as a defeat. Once I noticed halfway through a hike that I had forgotten to bring the ingenious device with me. Then it had all been for nothing."*
> *(J.P. Rawie, Dagblad van het Noorden, 10 April 2021: J.P. Rawie, Dutch weekly column in 'Newspaper of the North').*

Figure 1.
A quote from an AT user.

increase is a symptom that can indicate a (starting) inflammation/infection. Celsus, a Roman, already described "dolor, calor, tumor, and rubor" as inflammatory symptoms. And to date, not much has been added to that as "loss of function" as a symptom. Many nurses will be aware that these phenomena can occur when the deeper tissues in the foot are affected, in conjunction with nervous system abnormalities, neuropathies, and/or abnormalities of the blood vessels in the legs, and related angiopathies.

Diagnosis to prevent diabetic foot neuropathy (DFN) seems simple for professionals and relies on these historical principles. But it might become even easier for the patient using POCD: ask the person to use a measuring device (i.e., TempStat™) daily at home, more or less as if he were using a bathroom scale, but in this case, local heat is measured in the toes and sole of the foot. If a location the size of a pinhead with an elevated temperature is present, a message can be sent with a mobile phone to the general practitioner or nurse specialist, so that immediate action can be taken [8–10].

The thermal detection of phlebitis by using infrared techniques is an example of an innovation, currently in the experimental phase.

It is well known to clinical nurses that phlebitis is a common, painful complication of peripheral catheter infusion, occurring around the infusion needle insertion opening. Not only is it painful, but it can also lead to a longer hospital stay and even, rarely, death. The severity of phlebitis is currently scored using the "visual infusion phlebitis scale," the so-called (VIP) score, ranging from 0 (no phlebitis) to 5 (thrombophlebitis). In many cases, the scoring takes place when the damage has already been done and there is already an onset or already advanced thrombophlebitis at the time of the first measurement. Based on an experimental pilot study with expensive thermal cameras, which in principle were not developed for medical applications, thermal measurements were performed in adult I.C. patients (see **Figure 2**). A first pilot trial with relatively cheap smartphone applications shows that a very affordable and practical early thermal detection of ignition sources also seems possible. Further developments and trials will be needed before it will be possible to use the aforementioned camera's and measurement methods in practice [11].

4.4 Further developments related to POCD

What are the developments now and in the future in technological diagnostics? Out of many, the following are prominent promising examples:

1. *Hyperautomation technology* deals with the application of artificial intelligence (AI) and machine learning (ML) to increasingly (digitally) automate human processes. It concerns an intelligent form of robotization, in which self-learning computers (i.e., "avatars") continuously try to improve the results of their own

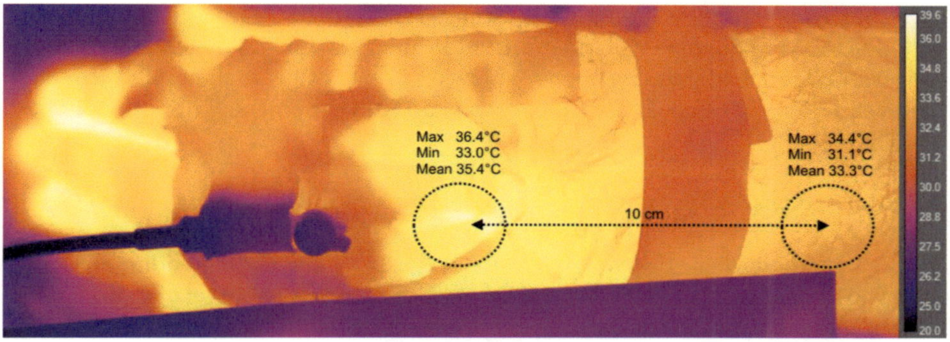

Figure 2.
Infrared image of a patient with a VIP 1 score. The maximum temperature at the insertion site (left circle) is 36.4°C and that of the proximal reference point (right circle) is 34.4°C. ΔT in this case is 2.0°C [11].

actions. "Babylon Health" is a well-known British company that mainly focuses on this [12].

2. *Multiexperience technology* abandons the traditional idea of a computer that has only a single point of interaction (i.e., a display). But it is based on multisensory and "multitouchpoint interfaces." This means that multiple interacting biosensors are linked to devices with which the results are presented attractively, such as wearables and the representation of (audible, tactile, and visible) results on trackers, watches, spectacle frames, and tablets. There are already many relatively simple applications on the Internet for this [13].

3. *Democratization technology* aims to make it easier for more and more people to become digitally skilled, and make the applications more "clunky," more intuitive, and more attractive for a wide audience, without the need for tedious, extensive explanation or training [14].

4. *Human augmentation*, in this context, is the use of technology to improve someone's cognitive and physical experiences, which can, for example, be used to increase the quality of the diagnostic process (i.e., to find an underlying reason for being inactive), with the aim to improve lifestyle more tailored (i.e., virtual 3D techniques) [15].

5. *Transparency and traceability technology* responds to the increasing responsibility, liability, and complexity in the safe, transparently ordered, usable, and findable storage of the ever-increasing amount of data of citizens (i.e., "e-patient movement") [16, 17].

6. *Haptic Tech*, or "kinesthetic communication," is the technology that allows the patient to relive the sense of touch through forces, vibrations, or movements in, for example, rehabilitation medicine [18].

7. *Fem Tech* (Female technology) is technology specifically aimed at women, such as fertility diagnostics, menstrual cycle tracking apps, and pregnancy monitoring [19].

8. *Swallowable Tech*: Sensors, such as "Smart-Pills," are oral capsules designed to collect data in the digestive tract for (additional) diagnostics such as local temperature and acid measurements. There are also capsule-shaped pills (partly in an experimental stage) that photograph and film the journey through the body [20, 21].

4.5 POCD and cost-effectiveness

Questions about cost-effectiveness (in the long run) when implementing POCD are not easy to answer scientifically. Because what is "quality of care" in relation to "efficiency in care provision"? What exactly do you measure that against? What is an acceptable gold standard? And in what (technological, professional) context is that valid?

The literature does talk about the way in which efficiency can be achieved by means of POCD; waiting times and lead time can be saved, as well as on transfers, reports, and other logistics processes: POCD could be more efficient.

It is hardly possible to find the scientific generalizability of a verifiable, workable, efficiency approach, on the basis of which demonstrable time and (financial) resources can be saved and where the quality of care is guaranteed. POCD could also be seen as a task burden. POCT can be added to the daily work practice of, for example, nurses, tests that were previously performed in the laboratory. It seems important in this context to look closely at adoption processes that can play a role in POCD [21–23].

4.6 Adoption of POCD

Implementing diagnostic technology does not happen by itself. Whether these will actually be used depends on several factors. The nature of the technological innovation, personal factors, team composition, and the degree of urgency that management attributes seem to play a role. The awareness that diagnostic technology has specific advantages for the patient, but could also lead to a reduction in the task—workload—of nurses, can be a positive influencing factor. This means that some diagnostic tests can offer a solution, not only to be able to diagnose quickly and efficiently so that you can act as a professional nurse, but also to be able to act appropriately on the basis of these quick and accurate results for use to immediate plan (preventive) actions to be carried out by the patient himself [22, 23].

Furthermore, the broad adoption of the aforementioned technology in regular general practice depends on many aspects. Other frequently mentioned influencing factors in the literature are:

- degree of familiarity (unknown makes unloved);
- costs (i.e., lack of clarity as to what reimbursement options are available with insurers);
- usability and user-friendliness (the essential success and failure factors);
- reliability (often only tested on the basis of "healthy standards");
- validity (once on the market, after the experimental phase, often made reasonably clear);

- safety (sometimes unclear to patients in specific situations. "*Can this be done with my pacemaker?*").
- compatibility (intelligently linked technological applications offer a broader diagnostic power compared to the (abovementioned) applications separately. This technology can, therefore, be used more cost-effectively) [20].

5. What should a POCD innovation contribute to?

Various recent government, industry, vision, and association reports state that technological innovations in general practice should contribute to two core values: "quality of life" and "affordability of care." This can, therefore, be seen as a qualitative and financial specification of the overarching objective: "accommodating the growing and changing demand for care." But, today, it does not stop there. Here is a "Top Ten" of frequently mentioned "innovation requirements" found in the various relevant reports.

5.1 A POCD innovation in general practice must

1. be effective (in terms of patient outcomes);
2. be efficient and sustainable (cost-effective and efficient);
3. not only serve the patient, but also "support the citizen in their social network";
4. allow the citizen (or the patient) and his/her immediate relatives to retain control (stimulation of self-management and joint management);
5. be wish-driven and demand-driven;
6. provide the citizen (or the patient) with information and knowledge in order to be able to use care in an appropriate and desired manner, and only if this is really necessary;
7. not only be used to diagnose diseases, but also for prevention and to improve lifestyle;
8. contribute to making the healthcare chain more transparent and accessible;
9. be safe (user safe and respect the legal frameworks regarding privacy);
10. be user-friendly for a (very) broad group of users [1–4, 21, 23].

6. Point-of-care internet diagnostics

The advent of technological diagnostics is no longer just a matter that concerns the healthcare professional. The patient or his immediate loved one will search for themselves if they cannot find a suitable answer to their question in regular care.

They find their way on digital patient forums, fellow sufferer forums, and the countless websites that present themselves as particularly reliable in diagnosing health problems. In any case, this development affects the practice of general practitioners. But the patient also comes to the specialist more often with Internet prior knowledge.

6.1 What is the quality of Internet diagnostics?

Few representative scientific results are known about medical diagnostic Internet services and what, for example, health effects, risks, and patient satisfaction are. According to these companies, which claim to be based on “years of best-practice experiences” and “scientifically substantiated action,” on average at least equivalent to a visit to a general practitioner, and sometimes even more reliable compared to the diagnoses and the advice obtained during a visit to the GP practice.

With techniques from artificial intelligence, the facial expression of the patient is also mapped and interpreted (is the conversation partner tense? Is there perhaps a question of pain?), whereby the self-learning ability of the systems used continues to reduce the margins of error. An app for transdermal blood analyzes is currently being worked on, and uploading the spectrum of a urine sample at home will also be an option. It is easy to guess what else the quantum computer can offer in the future [24–26].

6.2 A self-learning avatar

Is it not mostly advanced computer programs with extensive databases and search engines that do the work? Probably, at least to an increasing extent. Complaints that are relatively easy to understand are diagnosed by a friendly avatar in an unmistakable human guise; you can choose one that suits your preference: do you want to start a conversation with a man, a woman, an oriental, or a western appearance? The choice is yours. Photos of your skin, eyes, mucous membranes, etc. can provide additional diagnostic resources and can be uploaded immediately for review [24, 25, 27].

6.3 Commercial services in the diagnostic technology market

At the moment, (commercial) diagnostic service providers are appearing on the market who are happy to take work off the hands of the general practitioner and the nurse specialist. They even try to tempt the patient not to go to a general practice.

Advertisements in the form of YouTube films with street interviews in which citizens express their dissatisfaction with the travel time, poor accessibility, parking problems, waiting in the waiting room, the inconveniences they experience in the transfer of care, the problems in obtaining (repeat) prescriptions, the alleged dangers of contamination, going to the pharmacy with again long waiting times, etc. According to these stakeholders, it appears that a substantial part of the patients is ashamed of their own body and that they sometimes find it difficult to talk about personal problems in the consultation room, as a result of which they inadvertently create a barrier for themselves. These Internet services have the ultimate solution they proclaim themselves [24–26].

6.4 Diagnostic decision support systems

Whoever or whatever carries out the diagnostics, both the patient and the healthcare professional have an interest in the unambiguity and completeness of the diagnostic information and that it is only accessible in a legitimate form to those who, in good faith, want to know in an efficient manner taking this information.

It is very likely and hoped that the development of the current, rather limited functionality of the electronic file will be further developed into the so-called diagnostic decision support systems, which are supportive to both laymen and professionals. This development will continue for the time being on the basis of existing techniques (e.g., speech recognition, camera recognition, and artificial intelligence) and new (biometric) sensor applications. In the near future, patients will increasingly demand their data to search electronic systems and electronic forums around the world in order to obtain the very best solution for their health problems. Now you might be still—rightly—skeptical: "*So you are worried because you found something on the Internet that resembles what you might have?*"But perhaps the patient of the future will increasingly have an opinion that is similar to the conclusion you as a professional also draw. Certainly, if your own system will soon contain rich, reliable, logically ordered information and explanations, in that case, you may even want to stimulate your patient's digital search [15, 16, 28, 29].

7. Professional advice dilemma in POCD

A dilemma can arise if the introduction of a diagnostic application takes place via the patient. Increasingly, technology is presented to the physician by the patient or his close relative: "*Doctor, I found this device on the Internet, is something like this suitable for me?* "Diagnostic applications generally do not require a prescription and are widely available over the counter.

A nurse specialist who is well aware of recent technological diagnostic developments may be able to offer appropriate advice. But, unfortunately, there is no such thing as a repertory for the use of diagnostic technology, and a search for information will have to take place before really good advice can be given. [The database IEEE (ieee.org) does offer possibilities for quickly finding knowledge about diagnostic eHealth applications.]

7.1 Counseling dilemma

There could be a dilemma in providing information without the intervention of a healthcare professional, such as a physician or nurse specialist, if the diagnosis reveals a life-threatening, serious condition, for example. The traditional conversation, in which guidance with emotional information that has a major impact on life is central, may disappear in case of unguided, digital information gathering. Attention must be paid to this ethical dilemma. Being able to set up personal information filters could be a solution here. This does not alter the fact that professional, humane, compassionate guidance must always be available in case it is desired. The risk of POCD interfering with timely professional counseling and guidance should be avoided at all costs. In-depth qualitative and quantitative research to look specifically at these ethical aspects and to develop targeted interventions for this is, therefore, desirable. POCD should certainly also be followed from a philosophical point of view in this context.

7.2 The patient's appreciation of POCD

A lot will change in the service provision within healthcare in the coming years. A complete takeover by the healthcare avatar is not yet on the agenda, but it seems inevitable that it will acquire a place.

There are still some questions, concerns, and problems about "machine automated diagnostics" at the moment, such as legal issues, privacy issues, and ethical considerations (Is the provision of care still sufficiently "human," "patient-oriented," and "oriented to the entire social system"?)

The value that patients themselves attach to diagnostic possibilities (including Internet services) will determine its success. Insurers will be happy to join in on this.

Whether, for example, the nurse specialist and the general practitioner will eventually survive the technological revolution will depend, among other things, on whether they are also prepared to adopt POCD, QS techniques, and advanced Internet services, as digital services in many ways are expected to become an increasingly important part of healthcare procurement.

The promises are great. Before long, we will have arrived at automatic self-regulation, in which technical systems monitor, diagnose, and treat (semi) autonomously via noninvasive applications that are simply worn on the ankle.

Research, in that future juncture, will have to show whether it has ultimately contributed to the quality of life of many and aspects of healthy aging in general.

8. Conclusion

Point-of-care diagnostics will in all probability take off in a big way over the next 20–50 years. This will give many citizens the opportunity to monitor their own health accurately. In addition, it will increasingly provide automated information that helps prevent health risks. Increasing the compatibility of POCD applications with well-designed digital information systems over the chain of care, whereby the ease of use will be further amplified, shall be a necessary simultaneous development.

The further development of POCD will offer many possibilities for gathering knowledge by using new quantitative and qualitative research designs. Research, both on a phenomenological basis and on positivistic rounds in large samples, will support further professional development as well as enable citizens to make their own, well-informed choices. However, all these developments should never stand in the way of interpersonal, humane, and compassionate face-to-face care when it is really needed.

Author details

Wolter Paans[1,2]

1 Hanze University of Applied Sciences, Groningen, The Netherlands

2 Department of Critical Care, University Medical Centre Groningen, Groningen, The Netherlands

*Address all correspondence to: w.paans@pl.hanze.nl

References

[1] Lingervelder D, Koffijberg H, Emery JD, et al. How to realize the benefits of point of care testing at the general practice: A comparison of four high-income countries. International Journal of Health Policy and Management. 2021;**11**:2248-2260. DOI: 10.34172/ijhpm.2021.143

[2] Hopstaken RM, Kleinveld HA, van Balen JAM, Krabbe JG, van den Broek S, Weel J, et al. Richtlijn Point of care testing (POCT) in de huisartsenzorg. Nederlands Huisartsen Genootschap; 2015. Available from: https://research.utwente.nl/en/publications/richtlijn-point-of-care-testing-poct-in-de-huisartsenzorg

[3] Vashist SK. Point-of-care diagnostics: Recent advances and trends. Biosensors (Basel). 2017;**7**(4):62. DOI: 10.3390/bios7040062

[4] St John A, Price CP. Existing and emerging technologies for point-of-care testing. Clinical Biochemistry Reviews. 2014;**35**:155-167. Available from: http://www.ncbi.nlm.nih.gov/pmc/articles/PMC4204237/

[5] Paans W, Sprenger SR. How can activity trackers be useful? A scoping literature review. International Journal of Nursing and Health Care Research. 2022;**5**:1312. DOI: 10.29011/2688-9501.101312. Available from: www.gavinpublishers.com

[6] Cox EGM, Dieperink W, Wiersema R, Doesburg F, van der Meulen IC, Paans W. Temporal artery temperature measurements versus bladder temperature in critically ill patients, a prospective observational study. PLoS One. 2020;**15**(11):e0241846. DOI: 10.1371/journal.pone.0241846

[7] Mirwaes W, Besser M, e.a. Monitoring wound healing in a 3D wound model by hyperspectral imaging and efficient clustering. PLoS One. 2017;**12-12**:e0186425

[8] Houghton VJ, Bower VM, Chant DC. Is an increase in skin temperature predictive of neuropathic foot ulceration in people with diabetes? A systematic review and meta-analysis. Journal of Foot and Ankle Research. 2013;**6**(1):31. DOI: 10.1186/1757-1146-6-31

[9] Lazo-Porras M, Bernabe-Ortiz A, Sacksteder KA, Gilman RH, Malaga G, Armstrong DG, et al. Implementation of foot thermometry plus mHealth to prevent diabetic foot ulcers: Study protocol for a randomized controlled trial. Trials. 2016;**17**(1):206. DOI: 10.1186/s13063-016-1333-1

[10] Paans W. De diabetische voet: leidt bruikbare technologische zorgondersteuning tot zelfmanagement en zelfeffectiviteit? [The diabetic foot: does useful technological care support lead to self-management and self-efficacy?]. HuisartsenService, Medway. 2016;**5**(2):22-24. Available from: https://research.hanze.nl/ws/portalfiles/portal/24367177/Huisartsenservice_24_06_2016.pdf

[11] Doesburg F, Smit JM, Paans W, Onrust M, Nijsten MW, Dieperink W. Use of infrared thermography in the detection of superficial phlebitis in adult intensive care unit patients: A prospective single-center observational study. PLoS One. 2019;**14**(3):e0213754

[12] Peserico G, Morato A, Tramarin F, Vitturi S. Functional safety networks and protocols in the industrial internet of things era. Sensors (Basel). 2021;**21**(18):6073. DOI: 10.3390/s21186073

[13] Brudy F, Holz C, Rädle R, Wu C-J, Houben S, Klokmose CN, et al. Cross-device taxonomy: Survey, opportunities and challenges of interactions spanning across multiple devices. In: Proceedings of the 2019 CHI Conference on Human Factors in Computing Systems. Glasgow, United Kingdom: ACM/IEEE; 2019. DOI: 10.1145/3290605.3300792

[14] Wang Y, Yang B. Reinforcing health data sharing through data democratization. Studies in Health Technology and Informatics. 2021;**285**:124-129. DOI: 10.3233/SHTI210584

[15] Eden J, Bräcklein M, Ibáñez J, Barsakcioglu DY, Di Pino G, Farina D, et al. Principles of human movement augmentation and the challenges in making it a reality. Nature Communications. 2022;**13**(1):1345. DOI: 10.1038/s41467-022-28725-7

[16] deBronkart D, Eysenbach G. Gimme My Damn Data (and Let Patients Help!): The #GimmeMyDamnData Manifesto. Journal of Medical Internet Research. 2019;**21**(11):e17045. DOI: 10.2196/17045

[17] Lye CT, Forman HP, Gao R, Daniel JG, Hsiao AL, Mann MK, et al. Assessment of US hospital compliance with regulations for patients' requests for medical records. JAMA Network Open. 2018;**1**(6):e183014. DOI: 10.1001/jamanetworkopen.2018.3014

[18] Pineda R, Guth R, Herring A, Reynolds L, Oberle S, Smith J. Enhancing sensory experiences for very preterm infants in the NICU: An integrative review. Journal of Perinatology. 2017;**37**(4):323-332. DOI: 10.1038/jp.2016.179 Epub 2016 Oct 20

[19] Sandborg J, Söderström E, Henriksson P, Bendtsen M, Henström M, Leppänen MH, et al. Effectiveness of a smartphone app to promote healthy weight gain, diet, and physical activity during pregnancy (HealthyMoms): Randomized controlled trial. JMIR Mhealth and Uhealth. 2021;**9**(3):e26091. DOI: 10.2196/26091

[20] Paans W. De duurzaamheid van e-health toepassingen: een broos en complex samenspel, [The sustainability of e-health applications: A fragile and complex interplay]. HuisartsenService, MedWay. 2020;**9**(3):28-29 Available from: https://issuu.com/huisartsenservice/docs/_huisartsenservice_2020-3_online

[21] Golding MI, Doman DB, Goldberg HJ. Take your Pill(Cam): It might save your life. Gastrointestinal Endoscopy. 2005;**62**(1):196-198. DOI: 10.1016/s0016-5107(05)00543-2

[22] Lingervelder D, Koffijberg H, Kusters R, et al. Health economic evidence of point-of-care testing: A systematic review. Pharmaco-Economics Open. 2021;**5**:157-173. DOI: 10.1007/s41669-020-00248-1

[23] Vashist SK, Luppa PB, Yeo LY, Ozcan A, Luong JH. Emerging technologies for next-generation point-of-care testing. Trends in Biotechnology. 2015;**33**:692-705. DOI: 10.1016/j.tibtech.2015.09.001

[24] Peiffer-Smadja N, Rawson TM, Ahmad R, Buchard A, Georgiou P, Lescure FX, et al. Machine learning for clinical decision support in infectious diseases: A narrative review of current applications. Clinical Microbiology and Infection. 2020;**26**(5):584-595. DOI: 10.1016/j.cmi.2019.09.009. Epub 2019 Sep 17 [Erratum in: Clin Microbiol Infect. 2020;26(8):1118]

[25] Rizzo AA, Neumann U, Enciso R, Fidaleo D, Noh JY. Performance-driven

facial animation: Basic research on human judgments of emotional state in facial avatars. Cyberpsychology & Behavior. 2001;**4**(4):471-487. DOI: 10.1089/109493101750527033

[26] Kobie, N. Babylon disrupted the UK's health system. Then it left the AI-powered online doctor app is ditching its controversial NHS contracts as it focuses on the US market. Available from: https://www.wired.com/story/babylon-disrupted-uk-health-system-then-left/ (Posted 23 August 2022)

[27] Iacobucci G. Babylon health holds talks with "significant" number of NHS trusts. BMJ. 2020:m266. DOI: 10.1136/bmj.m266

[28] Groot, de K, Triemstra M, Paans W, Francke A. Quality criteria for nursing documentation: A systematic meta-review of systematic reviews. Journal of Advanced Nursing. 2018;**75**(7):1379-1393. DOI: 10.1111/jan.13919

[29] Müller-Staub M, de Graaf-Waar H, Paans W. An internationally consented standard for nursing process-clinical decision support systems in electronic health records. Computers, Informatics, Nursing. 2016;34(11):493-502. DOI: 10.1097/CIN.0000000000000277

Chapter 9

Global Critical Shortage of Nurses: Pathway to Solution

Almas Bandeali and Zeeba Maita

Abstract

In 2020, the first State of the World's Nursing (SOWN) report published by the World Health Organization (WHO) revealed global nursing workforce to be at 27.9 million. SOWN estimated a current global nursing shortfall of 5.9 million. Furthermore, 17% of nurses are expected to retire in next 10 years. An estimated 5.3 million (89%) of that shortage is concentrated in low and lower-middle income countries, where the growth in the number of nurses is barely keeping pace with population growth. WHO global Strategic Directions for Nursing and Midwifery (SDNM) 2022 report has identified policy focus interventions for four major areas: education, jobs, leadership, and service delivery. Nurse advocacy groups like International Council of Nurses (ICN) are calling on governments to partner with various healthcare stakeholders to find tangible solutions in addressing global nursing shortage (NS).

Keywords: nursing shortage, global nursing crisis, global nursing disparities, nursing shortage an ethical concern, nursing supply strategies, nursing policies and practices

1. Introduction

Our world is one society at large, woven in one fabric of causation. What happens in one end of our world impacts us all. Coronavirus disease 2019 (COVID-19) pandemic has certainly affirmed, we as global community are only as stronger as our weakest link [1–5]. Having to manage exhausted health care workers (HCWs), supply chain limitations, and budgeting constrains from an economic meltdown, healthcare organizations are battling a 'perfect storm' in staying afloat. If the foundation of a structure is weak, that structure is bound to collapse in due time. Inability to protect our HCWs is analogous to failed health care systems. COVID-19 pandemic has been a catalyst in understanding the gaps in our healthcare ecosystem, hence an opportunity to fix them [6]. This chapter will attempt to discuss current dialogs, development of trends, and limitations among various actors in managing global critical shortage of nurses. Lastly, the authors will share their constructive implications for NS from a holistic lens.

2. Body: nurses - the building blocks of our healthcare ecosystem

For Healthcare industry, it is fundamental to ensure that patients receive a superior experience when journeying through their facilities. Face-to-face between

IntechOpen

HCWs and patients is the path forward for safe and efficient patient-centred care. In a world that is already facing dramatic shortage of HCWs, WHO estimates an additional 18 million HCWs will be needed in the next decade [2, 7, 8]. Although, every HCW is essential in maintaining a functional healthcare system, in that, nurses are the 'building blocks' of any healthcare organization. There is a shift in power dynamics within the healthcare space from doctor being the pinnacle of primary care to patients and their nurse advocates gaining autonomy in practicing patient centred care. Nurses are the gatekeepers to patient engagement, spending more time with patients than any other HCW and patient experience satisfaction is highly dependent on these interactions [9].

3. Global critical nurse shortage

Healthcare industry was tackling global NS even before the pandemic. In 2020, WHO published SOWN report that highlights global nursing workforce to be 27.9 million, estimating 5.9 million NS globally [1].

The report indicates, 89% NS is concentrated in low-income and lower-middle-income WHO countries (Africa, South-East Asia, and Eastern Mediterranean) [2, 3]. Globally, 17% nurses are expected to retire in the next 10 years, needing to educate and employe 4.7 million nurses to only maintain current workforce numbers, without addressing the shortage [5]. In total, 10.6 million nurses will be needed by 2030 [3].

4. United Nations sustainable developmental goals

In 2015, United Nations (UN) Member States provided 17 Sustainable Developmental Goals (SDGs) to be achieved in global partnership, by all countries-developed and developing for peace and prosperity for all people and the planet, now and into the future [10]. Health worker density and distribution is indicator 3.c.1 of the UN SDGs, helping to track recruitment, development, training, and retention of healthcare workforce [10, 11]. In 2019, a systematic analysis for the global burden of disease (GBD) study measuring the availability of human resources for health (HRH) and its relationship to universal health coverage (UHC) for 204 countries and territories from 1990 to 2019 indicated, the world had 104·0 million (95% uncertainty interval 83·5–128·0) HCWs including 12·8 million (9·7–16·6) physicians, 29·8 million (23·3–37·7) nurses and midwives, 4·6 million (3·6–6·0) dentistry personnel, and 5·2 million (4·0–6·7) pharmaceutical personnel [11]. A global physician density of 16·7 (12·6–21·6) per 10,000 population, and a nurse and midwife density of 38·6 (30·1–48·8) per 10,000 population, was calculated [11]. GBD super-regions of sub-Saharan Africa, south Asia, north Africa, and the Middle East had the lowest HRH densities [11]. To reach 80 out of 100 on the UHC effective coverage index, an estimation per 10,000 population, at least 20·7 physicians, 70·6 nurses and midwives, 8·2 dentistry personnel, and 9·4 pharmaceutical personnel would be needed [11]. In total, the 2019 national health workforces fell short of these minimum thresholds by 6·4 million physicians, *30·6 million nurses and midwives*, 3·3 million dentistry personnel, and 2·9 million pharmaceutical personnel [11].

5. Gap broadens with COVID-19

Two-thirds (66%) WHO Member States report pandemic related disruption to health services due to factors related to HCWs [12]. COVID-19 has been devastating on all HCWs but especially nurses who have been front and center, managing heavy workload, long hours with maximum exposure to coronavirus, while caring for their patients. They will remain the mainstay profession in the recovery of post-COVID-19 health systems, even though it comes at a terrible cost of their overall well-being [5, 13]. WHO acknowledges, all though a "conservative" number due to underreporting, 115, 500 HCWs lost their lives because of COVID-19 [12]. Many nurses have died, others are mentally burnout, and many more continue to suffer physically; victims of long-haul COVID-19 syndrome because of poor provision of personal protective equipment (PPE) and inadequate access to vaccines [12, 13].

6. Nurse shortage - a multilayered complex problem

To fully articulate a solution means to consider the gaps and shortfalls in the political, social, economic, and institutional realities on and through which this issue is constructed. For example, if we only consider NS as a problem of numbers – then the temporary fix will be producing more nurses. If the shortage is associated towards nurses being dissatisfied with their working environment – then improvements in their work environment resolves that problem only. Only addressing these problems in isolation is merely a short-term fix and will result in relapse. Upon the request of 73rd World Health Assembly (WHA), WHO engaged with all WHO regions and updated global SDNM 2016–2020 to SDNM 2021–2025 in resolution with 74th WHA for NS policy action [4]. "To identify the most important policy actions, a prioritization exercise was conducted with over 600 nursing and midwifery leaders from ministries of health, national nursing and midwifery associations, regulators, WHO collaborating centres for nursing and midwifery, and the Nursing Now campaign in attendance at the biennial WHO global forum of Government Chief Nursing and Midwifery Officers and at the 'Triad' meeting hosted by WHO, the International Confederation of Midwives, and the International Council of Nurses. Regional and global consultation processes corroborated and helped refine the prioritized policies. The policy priorities are interrelated: the issues and policy responses in one are correlated with the issues and policy responses in the others" [4].

7. Pathway to solution

7.1 SDNM encompasses four areas

Education, jobs, leadership, and service delivery, for strategic direction [4]. Each area comprising of two to four prioritized policy actions are collectively interrelated and interdependent (**Table 1**).

EDUCATION →	JOBS →
Strategic direction: Midwife and nurse graduates match or surpass health system demand and have the requisite knowledge, competencies and attitudes to meet national health priorities.	Strategic direction: Increase the availability of health workers by sustainably creating nursing and midwifery jobs, effectively recruiting and retaining midwives and nurses, and ethically managing international mobility and migration.
Policy priority: Align the levels of nursing and midwifery education with optimized roles within the health and academic systems.	Policy priority: Conduct nursing and midwifery workforces planning and forecasting through a health labour market lens.
Policy priority: Optimize the domestic production of midwives and nurses to meet or surpass health system demand.	Policy priority: Ensure adequate demand (jobs) with respect to health service delivery for primary health care and other population health priorities.
Policy priority: Design education programmes to be competency-based, apply effective learning design, meet quality standards, and align with population health needs.	Policy priority: Reinforce implementation of the WHO Global Code of Practice on the International Recruitment of Health Personnel.
Policy priority: Ensure that faculty are properly trained in the best pedagogical methods and technologies, with demonstrated clinical expertise in content areas.	Policy priority: Attract, recruit and retain midwives and nurses where they are most needed.
LEADERSHIP →	SERVICE DELIVERY →
Strategic direction: Increase the proportion and authority of midwives and nurses in senior health and academic positions and continually develop the next generation of nursing and midwifery leaders.	Strategic direction: Midwives and nurses work to the full extent of their education and training in safe and supportive service delivery environments.
Policy priority: Establish and strengthen senior leadership positions for nursing and midwifery workforce governance and management and input into health policy.	Policy priority: Review and strengthen professional regulatory systems and support capacity building of regulators, where needed.
Policy priority: Invest in leadership skills development for midwives and nurses.	Policy priority: Adapt workplaces to enable midwives and nurses to maximally contribute to service delivery in interdisciplinary health care teams.
Global strategic directions for nursing and midwifery 2021–2025.	

Table 1.
WHO (2021). Global Strategic Directions for Nursing and Midwifery (SDNM) 2021–2025 [4].

7.2 Nurse practitioners as primary care providers

One strategy being utilized in decreasing healthcare cost is to expand the scope of practice by shifting the delivery of treatment management to nurses. In 2015, Nebraska became the 20th state to adopt a law that allows nurses with advanced degrees to practice particular medical fields without a doctor's oversight [9]. The law helps rural areas that have trouble recruiting physicians but have high healthcare need due to aging populations to still provide care through nurse practitioners (NPs). "According to the Institute of Medicine, 14 NPs can be trained for the cost of a single physician, and research shows that primary care outcomes by NPs is equivalent to that of physicians" [9]. What this boils down to, evidence based research shows that, for certain forms of primary care, NPs are not only more cost-efficient by providing better value to the healthcare system but have also reduced morbidity and mortality when caring for vulnerable (aging, rural) population [9, 14–16].

7.3 Nurse shortage: "quick fix" recruitments a need for policy reform

Pre-pandemic NS along with pandemic has increased the demand for "fast-tack" international nurse recruitment by some high-income Organization for Economic Co-operation and Development (OECD) countries, which could undermine the ability of some "source" countries to respond effectively to pandemic challenges [17]. Even before the pandemic, the scale of the international flow of nurses was large, and growing. In 2019, OECD analysis highlighted more than 550,000 foreign-trained nurses were working across 36 OECD member countries, which was a marked increase on the 460,000 recorded in 2011 [17]. OECD reports the number and/or share of foreign-trained nurses has increased particularly rapidly in Belgium, France, Germany and Switzerland, with a steady growth also occurring in Australia, New Zealand, Canada [18] and the United States [17]. SOWN highlighted that countries experiencing low densities of nurses are mostly located in the WHO African, South-East Asia and Eastern Mediterranean regions, and in parts of Latin America, with countries accounting for the largest shortages (in numerical terms) in 2018 included Bangladesh, India, Indonesia, Nigeria, and Pakistan only to be worsened with population growth [1, 17]. In 2020, World Bank Group study examining nurse labour markets in countries (Botswana, Eswatini, Kenya, Lesotho, Malawi, Mauritius, Mozambique, Namibia, Rwanda, Seychelles, South Africa, South Sudan, Tanzania, Uganda, Zambia, Zimbabwe) of the Eastern, Central and Southern African (ESCA) region reported, that demand for nurses was growing, but high vacancy rates (30–55%) in the public sector remained a problem [19]. Nurses do not fill posts due to "poor wage, remote location, lack of amenities, and poor working conditions" [19]. Additionally, the ECSA study highlighted, by 2030, 4.7 billion dollars would be required to train additional nurses to achieve the number needed in the 14 countries alone [19].

To adjust the supply and demand disproportion, international policy actors will require to reinforce policies upon OECD countries that lure nurses from low-income and lower-middle income countries. There is a growing policy emphasis on the potential of government- to- government bilateral agreements to "manage" international recruitment of nurses — these agreements must be independently monitored to assure full compliance by all parties [17]. Simultaneously, countries will need to invest an extra ~1% of GDP in their health workforce, as part of a broader investment package to boost health system resilience; basing this estimate on benchmarking analysis to estimate additional health workers, higher salaries, and medical reserve needed, said the head of health division at OECD in a presentation to the ICN Congress [20, 21]. Furthermore, one of the most powerful policy levers governments can use to adjust the supply of doctors and nurses to projected demand is so-called *numerus clausus*, that is, the regulation of the number of students entering medical and nursing education programmes; as in several OECD countries, *numerus clausus* policies are still based on weak evidence and opaque decision-making processes [20].

8. Conclusion

The need for collectively intervention with short and long term shared action plan is imminent in supporting global crisis of nurse shortage. Recurrence of NS overtime is perhaps a testament for a more beneficial analysis to address a complex issue, including many overlapping and interconnected problems from a global platform. As advocated by international actors that influence nursing policies and practices, there is an overall need to invest in nursing education, jobs, leadership, and service delivery to meet the demand and maintain a steady supply of nurses [2, 3, 17].

The authors recommend following implementations:

1. Global standardization of nursing education – to provide cultural holistic care of the populations served in practice, due to vast migration and immigration trends.

2. Creating a central, open access education database of nursing best practices – to standardize general concepts and care; reduce duplication by central sharing of resources; osmosis of academic knowledge exchange enhances and increases mobility of data. Education needs to keep up with globalization.

3. International provision for student nurses from all countries to participate in clinical exchange programs – currently nursing programs in developing countries allow international students from similar caliber institutions to participate in an exchange program; however, such opportunities do not exist for nursing students enrolled in programs 'less visible' from lack of funding and/or their geo-political standings. A student nurses' color of passport or their.

4. A global hub for nursing licensure model – to facilitate mobility of sustainable best-practices for retention among countries.

5. National nursing bodies to hold a political seat in their respective ministry of health portfolios – collaboration on a political platform will enhance and enforce sustainable, constructive, inclusive, relevant policies and practices from, macro (national/governance), meso (institutional/academic), and micro (community/clinical) levels.

6. Offer standardized specialty nursing and NP programs – to meet the demand of primary care providers needed along with meeting the needs to care for patients in a specialized medical setting, which is becoming more-and-more norm of our healthcare ecosystem.

Without sufficient well-motivated and supported nurses, the global health system cannot function. A co-ordinated policy response at country level and internationally is urgently needed to improve nurse retention and give hope for the future sustainability of the nursing profession [17].

Author contributions

AB is the primary author, ZM is the co-author who partnered after the abstract was approved by the editors; Collectively, AB and ZM collaborated to revise and develop the search criteria, completed the initial search for the manuscript, and assessed articles for inclusion criteria; AB wrote the initial draft of the manuscript; ZM edited that draft; AB and ZM collectively finalized the final manuscript for submission.

Conflict of interests

The authors declare that there is no conflict of interest.

Acronyms

COVID-19	Coronavirus disease 2019
ECSA	Eastern, Central, and Southern African
GBD	Global burden of disease
HCWs	Health care workers
HRH	Human resources for health
ICN	International Council of Nurses
NHWA	National Health Workforce Accounts
NS	Nursing/Nurse shortage
NPs	Nurse practitioners
OECD	Organization for Economic Co-operation and Development
PPE	Personal protective equipment
SOWN	State of the World's Nursing
SDNM	Strategic Directions for Nursing and Midwifery
SDGs	Sustainable Development Goals
UN	United Nations
UHC	Universal health coverage
WHA	World Health Assembly
WHO	World Health Organization

Author details

Almas Bandeali[1*] and Zeeba Maita[2]

1 United Nations Interreginal Crime and Justice Research Institute, Italy

2 York University, Canada

*Address all correspondence to: almas.bandeali@graduateinstitute.ch

References

[1] World Health Organization. State of the world's nursing 2020: Investing in education, jobs and leadership. 2020. Retrieved September 10, 2022. Available from: https://www.who.int/publications/i/item/9789240003279

[2] World Health Organization. State of world's nursing 2020: Investing in education, jobs, and leadership. Retrieved online from National Health Workforce Accounts (NHWA) data base. 2021. Retrieved September 10, 2022. Available from: https://apps.who.int/nhwaportal/Home/Index

[3] International Council of Nurses. The global nursing shortage and nurse retention. Retrieved September 8, 2022. 2021. Available from: https://www.icn.ch/sites/default/files/inline-files/ICN%20Policy%20Brief_Nurse%20Shortage%20and%20Retention.pdf

[4] World Health Organization. Global strategic directions for nursing and midwifery (SDNM) 2021-2025. 2021. Retrieved September 10, 2022. Available from: https://www.who.int/publications/i/item/9789240033863

[5] Stewart D et al. Nurses: A voice to lead. In: Invest in Nursing and Respect Rights to Global Health. Geneva: International Council of Nurses. Retrieved September 19, 2022; 2022. Available from: https://www.icn.ch/system/files/2022-10/ICN_IND_Toolkit_English_FINAL.pdf

[6] World Health Organization. Working for health and growth: Investing in the health workforce. In: High-Level Commission on Health Employment and Economic Growth. Geneva: WHO; 2016. Retrieved September 15, 2022. Available from: https://apps.who.int/iris/bitstream/handle/10665/250047/9789241511308-eng.pdf

[7] Talisuna A et al. The urgent need for a global commitment to protect healthcare workers. BMJ Global Health. 2020;**5**:e004077. Retrieved October 01, 2022. Available from: https://gh.bmj.com/content/bmjgh/5/11/e004077.full.pdf

[8] Protecting health care workers: A need for urgent action. NY, USA: Resolve to save lives. Retrieved September 29, 2022. 2021. Available from: https://preventepidemics.org/covid19/resources/protecting-hcw/

[9] Aita J, Johnston-Jewell D, Lobb R. The fall of the doctor and the rise of the nurse. Canadian Medical Association Journal, January 2021. 2019:41-44. Retrieved January 2021 from hardcopy subscription

[10] United Nations. 2015. Transforming our world: the 2030 agenda for Sustainable Development Goals. General Assembly: A/RES/70/1. Retrieved February 2018. Available from: https://documents-dds-ny.un.org/doc/UNDOC/GEN/N15/291/89/PDF/N1529189.pdf?OpenElement

[11] Lozano R et al. Measuring the availability of human resources for health and its relationship to universal health coverage for 204 countries and territories from 1990 to 2019: A systematic analysis for the global burden of disease study 2019. Lancet. 2019;**399**:2129-2154. Retrieved October 22, 2022. Available from: https://www.thelancet.com/pdfs/journals/lancet/PIIS0140-6736(22)00532-3.pdf

[12] World Health Organization. The impact of COVID-19 on health and care

workers: A closer look at deaths. Health Workforce Department – Working Paper 1. 2021. Retrieved March 21, 2022. Available from: https://apps.who.int/iris/bitstream/handle/10665/345300/WHO-HWF-WorkingPaper-2021.1-eng.pdf?sequence=1&isAllowed=y

[13] Galanis P et al. Nurses' burnout and associated risk factors during the COVID-19 pandemic: A systematic review and meta-analysis. Journal of Advanced Nursing. 2021;**77**:3286-3302. Retrieved October 29, 2022. Available from: https://www.ncbi.nlm.nih.gov/pmc/articles/PMC8250618/pdf/JAN-77-3286.pdf

[14] Moaven R et al. Drivers of cost differences between nurse practitioner and physician attributed medicare beneficiaries. Medical Care. 2021;**59**(2):177-184. Retrieved September 28, 2022. Available from: https://journals.lww.com/lww-medicalcare/Fulltext/2021/02000/Drivers_of_Cost_Differences_Between_Nurse.13.aspx

[15] Martínez-González et al. Substitution of physicians by nurses in primary care: A systematic review and meta-analysis. BMC Health Services Research. 2014;**14**:214. Retrieved October 04, 2022. Available from: https://www.ncbi.nlm.nih.gov/pmc/articles/PMC4065389/pdf/1472-6963-14-214.pdf

[16] Speight C et al. Strategies to promote the professional transition of new graduate nurse practitioners: A systematic review. Journal of Nursing Forum. 2019;**54**:557-564. Retrieved October 04, 2022. Available from: https://www.nppostgradtraining.com/wp-content/uploads/2020/08/transition-to-practice-1-Copy.pdf

[17] Buchan J, Catton H, Shaffer F. The global nursing workforce and the COVID19 pandemic. In: International Centre on Nurse Migration. Retrieved September 27, 2022. 2022. Available from: https://www.icn.ch/system/files/2022-01/Sustain%20and%20Retain%20in%202022%20and%20Beyond-%20The%20global%20nursing%20workforce%20and%20the%20COVID-19%20pandemic.pdf

[18] Advisory Committee on Health Human Resources. Our health, our future. Creating quality workplaces for Canadian nurses. In: The Canadian Nursing Advisory Committee. Ottawa: Government of Canada. Retrieved September 13, 2022; 2002. Available from: https://www.canada.ca/en/health-canada/services/health-care-system/reports-publications/nursing/health-future-creating-quality-workplaces-canadian-nurses-final-report-canadian-nursing.html

[19] World Bank Group. Eastern, Central, and Southern African Region education and labor markets for nurses: Challenges and opportunities. 2021. Retrieved October 04, 2022. Available from: https://www.icn.ch/sites/default/files/inline-files/WBG_ECSA%5B12%5D.pdf

[20] Organization for Economic Co-operation and Development. Health workforce policies: Right jobs, right skills, right places, Chapter 3: Education and training for doctors and nurses: What's happening with numerus clausus policies? Retrieved September 29, 2022. 2016. Available from: https://www.oecd-ilibrary.org/docserver/9789264239517-6-en.pdf?expires=1669598840&id=id&accname=guest&checksum=F9F3C3F7770D318FB07FFB3EC1B56144

[21] Colombo F. Investing in nurses and other health workers is an investment in health system resilience. In: Presentation to ICN Congress. Geneva, Switzerland: ICN. Retrieved September 13, 2022. 2021. Available from: https://icncongress2021.org/uploads/2021/10/Congress_Guide_DRAFT_V9.pdf

Chapter 10

Nurse Prescribing

Hamidreza Haririan

Abstract

Nurses, as the most numerous human resources in the field of health, have many roles and responsibilities. The number of countries where nurse prescribing is common is increasing. Also, the legal, educational, and organizational conditions in which a nurse prescribes medication vary greatly from country to country, ranging from the fact that the nurse can only prescribe from a limited list and under the supervision of a physician to the case where the nurse is authorized to prescribe without any restrictions. In many countries, health policymakers have responded to increasing demand for care due to aging populations and the increasing prevalence of chronic disease, physician shortages, and budget constraints, through strategies such as modernizing roles and combining health professions, including the role development of nurses. Prescribing by nurses has been a historic move for the nursing profession and an important part of the health system solution in leading countries to improve access and reduce the waiting time for patients to receive medication. Other potential benefits of nurse prescribing are increased continuity of patient care and better access to medication, efficiency in drug delivery and patient comfort, and reduced patient waiting time.

Keywords: authority, cost effective, health service, nurse, prescription

1. Introduction

Nurses have different roles in the health system and these roles can be changed or revised according to the needs of the society and increasing the ability of nurses [1]. Nurse prescribing is considered as the one of the new roles in the world, the implementation of which requires knowledge, skill, and clinical experience in nurses [2]. Written or oral prescribing requires complex and challenging skills. According to the Oregon Nurse Practice Act, nurse prescribing refers to the process in which a nurse recommends medication or dispenses medicines for patients [3].

Although nurse prescribing was first done in 1986 in the UK, in recent years, evidence of a significant development in the role of nurse prescribing has been seen in various countries, for example, in countries such as South Africa, Ireland, Canada, Norway, Netherlands, Sweden, Spain, and USA, nurses have the legal right to prescribe [4]. The legal, educational, and organizational conditions in which a nurse prescribes medication vary greatly from country to country. A nurse may only be allowed to prescribe from a limited list of medications under the supervision of a physician to being authorized to prescribe without any restrictions [5]. Nurses' ability to prescribe has been a historic development for the profession and an important part of the solution in many health systems in leading countries to improve access and reduce the waiting time for patients to receive medication [6].

In England, for the first time in 1986, the nurse prescription was proposed by the British Health Department, in such a way that nurses assessed the patients and after diagnosing the problem, they waited for the physician to confirm and stamp the diagnosis and prescription taken by the nurse. In 1989, in the first report of the Crown, the prescription of nurses within a specific pharmaceutical range was supported, and in 1998, the nurse prescription from the list of drugs (Nurse prescribers formulary) was approved nationally in the United Kingdom, and based on the opinion of the government, in 2000, nurse prescription was developed and the drug list with more scope became official with the title (Extend nurse prescribers formulary) [7]. And finally in 2006 the independent prescription of drugs from the British national formulary became official and the registered nurses who had at least 3 years of work experience were allowed to participate in prescription training courses. According to the drug list of 2002, nurse prescribers in the United Kingdom prescribed 180 drugs for about 80 clinical conditions, which reached 240 drugs for 110 different clinical situations in 2005, and since 2006, nurse prescribers could prescribe all authorized drugs except for some restricted drugs including special narcotics [8].

In some countries, prescription laws are exclusive and include physicians and nurse practitioners. The United States of America is one of these countries, and in some states, optometrists, psychologists, and nurses with special clinical experience can also prescribe within the specified limits. Nurse Practitioners were able to obtain a prescription license for the first time in 1969 in the United States, and in 2004, they started prescribing drugs in about 40 American states [7]. It should be noted that in some countries, nurse prescription is being implemented in clinical areas such as chronic diseases, cystic fibrosis, diabetes, cardiovascular disease, general surgery and pain control, renal failure, and substance abuse [9].

There are many reasons for endorsing prescribing rights to nurses including the following: improving the quality of medical care delivery, reducing treatment time and expense, increasing nurses' job independence, and helping nurses to make better use of their professional skills [2]. The right to prescribe can enhance nurses' sense of independence, usefulness, and professionalism [10]. The purpose of prescribing in nursing is not to turn a nurse into a physician, but to increase health in the community, especially in basic and primary care, which can enable the level of access and cheaper services. Nurse prescribing can bring the following advantages: timely, rapid, and convenient access of patients to medication, treatment, and care (especially in chronic diseases), reduced patients waiting time, improved efficiency of care and medical services, constant and extensive prescriber-patient communication, optimal use of nurses, patients, and physicians' time, engagement of nurses in non-repetitive and non-routine tasks, better control of disease symptoms, reducing the number of admissions and length of stay, and reduced health costs [2, 11]. Since cost containment is one of the main policies of health systems in countries, the government officials consider changing duties and roles and assigning some tasks from physicians to nurses as one of the important ways. In addition, the nursing profession has developed strategies to increase the advancement of the nursing profession, increasing autonomy with introduction of specialized roles that include nurses having prescribing rights [4].

In specialist wards, such as the Intensive Care Unit (ICU) and the Cardiac Care Unit (CCU), due to the nature of the ward and the acuity of the patients, nurses have more scientific and practical capabilities that lead to clinically competent nursing staff. Also, due to the critical condition of the patient, it is sometimes necessary for nurses to make quick and sudden decisions to save the patient's life, among which one of these decisions may be prescribing medication or other life-saving care measures that ultimately improve patient outcomes [12].

The World Health Organization (WHO) discussed the role of nurses and their performance in prescribing in different countries in the consultative panel of the Eastern Mediterranean Region Nursing Forum in 2001 and considered them ready to prescribe medicine. However, the prescription by the nurse, like the prescription by the physicians, can include drug side effects, wrong diagnosis, or incorrect prescription [13].

Nurse prescribing in some countries for example in Iran is in its infancy, because there have only been discussions in this regard and no executive action has been taken so far, and it is clear that giving this duty to nurses in these countries requires providing the necessary conditions such as creating preparation and increasing the authority of nurses [10]. Darvishpour [14] conducted a qualitative study entitled nurse prescribing in Iran and abroad. She reported that, despite the public assumption that nurse prescribing is not practiced in Iran, it is carried out in most wards, especially in emergency departments and intensive care units. In addition, like other countries, there are independent and dependent prescribing practices, but the quality and manner of prescribing is greatly different in Iran because nurse prescribing is carried out illegally and, in some cases, secretly [14]. In the study by Babaie et al. [15] that aimed to determine the attitude and readiness of Iranian nurses toward nurse prescribing, the results showed that nurses had a good preparation and attitude toward nurse prescribing [15].

2. Nurse prescribing challenges

Worldwide, there are challenges to nurse prescribing, which include the following:

1. **The critical view of the health care team** due to the lack of trust between nurses and physicians and the opposition of physicians to the approval and legalization of nurse prescriptions [16].

2. **The lack of support for nurses** from the authorities, leaving daily medical tasks to nurses, and hierarchical norms and strict control of nurses by physicians contrary to legal regulations [16].

3. **Failure to pay attention to the assessment of professional competence** due to the limitations of scientific and specialized knowledge of nurses and their lack of pharmacology knowledge [17]. Of course, these problems can be solved by continuously evaluating and monitoring the clinical competence of nurses, increasing the level of pharmacology knowledge, holding specialized courses, and having at least 3 years of work experience and participating in training courses [18].

4. **The legal restrictions** of prescribing by nurses [19].

5. **The public's lack of awareness** of the role of nurse prescribers [20].

In the beginning, some countries, including Britain, had a negative view of prescription other than physicians, and the passage of time and the favorable performance of nurses have been effective in modulating this view [21]. Today, nurse prescription policies are different in countries; for example, in US, several years after the legalization of the role of nurse prescription, it is still associated with the opposition of physicians, which has led to a lack of trust between nurses and physicians [16]. Some physicians, regardless of the positive aspect of nurse prescription and full knowledge, consider this role to be the handing over of routine medical work to nursing and are against increasing the authority of nurses in prescribing and believe that the expansion of this role is based on hierarchical norms or the same view. From top to bottom, it undermines that the physician is always at the top of decision making and the nurses are the ones who execute their orders, which has resulted in unfair strictures in nursing prescriptions [22].

Carey and colleagues [23] consider the lack of cooperation and support of the health care team in clinical management programs to be the problem of supplementary prescribing by nurses [23]. Other problems in the field of nurse prescription include the lack of government support in terms of finances and budget allocation, the lack of cooperation of insurances with nursing prescriptions and neglect of the training of prescribing nurses, as well as the lack of support of nurses from each other and the limited number of training courses [8]. Increasing the knowledge and expertise of nurses, increasing teamwork, supporting each other's colleagues, clinical supervision by the supervisor and continuous professional development, and increasing the support of officials are mentioned as suitable ways to reduce and solve this challenge [24].

Failure to pay attention to the evaluation of the professional qualifications of nurses will cause irreparable damage to health care system. According to Afseth and Paterson's study [25], it is very important to pay attention to the way of practice in the examination of professional competence, and the clarification of professional qualifications should be done in nurse prescription before designing and prescribing permission to nurses through the participation of stakeholders [25]. Qualification criteria for nurses are important in relation to pharmacology knowledge and drug calculations, which is one of the most important qualifications required for independent nursing prescription, having at least 3 years of clinical work experience and participating in specialized training courses [18].

According to Ax's study [26], weakness in drug calculations and inaccuracy in determining the appropriate drug dosage are one of the obstacles to obtaining a legal license in nursing prescription. Careful training of nurses solves the problem to a large extent. Many pharmaceutical companies have solved the problem of complex pharmaceutical calculation in new pharmaceutical products [26]. In all the countries where there is a nursing prescription, nurses need to pass a special training course for a drug prescription in order to be allowed to prescribe medicine [27]. In the UK, there is no specific course required to prescribe a Patient Group Guide (PGD). The training course and the conditions and qualifications required for prescribing nursing are different in different countries; for example in Australia, US, Canada, and New Zealand, nurses are required to be allowed to prescribe medicine independently before completing advanced nursing education, while in Ireland and England this condition is not required and nurses in the United Kingdom have the right to prescribe widely [28]. Also, the criteria for entering the drug prescribing period by nurses in different countries are different, so in England it is at least 3 years of work experience, in New Zealand 4 years, and in Australia 5 years [28].

Competencies and nursing training courses in England include a 39-day period, which lasts 3 to 6 months. This course includes 27 days of theory and 12 days of internship, which is done under the supervision of a mentor. The theory part can be presented remotely and in its own way. The things that are studied in the nursing training program are as follows: (1) psychological and therapeutic effects of the nurse prescribing, (2) counseling, decision making, treatment, and referral, (3) prescribing within a team context, (4) clinical pharmacology and complications, (5) evidence-based care, (6) legal and ethical aspects of prescribing, (7) professional responsibility and accountability, and (8) prescribing in the public health. The practical part and internship, which is done very strictly and accurately, includes the OSCE functional test and the final exam of pharmacology and its use in practice [29].

In many countries, nurse prescribing is associated with legal restrictions, and usually, nurses are allowed to prescribe drugs that are OTC or are allowed to prescribe from a specified list of drugs [21]. The opposition of physicians to the approval of this role, the lack of familiarity of policymakers with non-medical prescription, and fear of making mistakes in the opinion of nurses are mentioned as the reasons for legal restriction [16]. However, according to the study by Carberry et al. [30] an audit in the prescriptions of nurse practitioners (Advanced Nurse Practitioners in Critical Care) was done. And out of 388 drugs prescribed by nurses only 2 errors (0.6%) were found, while, in relation to physicians out of 984 drugs 32 errors (3.4%) were found. Based on the results of this audit, the error score was significantly different between groups, and the highest error score was related to physicians [30].

From the past, nursing has had the appearance of being dependent on physician as an executor of physician's orders, and this issue has been very confusing for nurses and has weakened social identity and public trust. By increasing the professional independence of nurses, it is hoped that these pressures will be reduced. According to Grad et al.'s study [20], due to a lack of knowledge about the nurse prescribing, despite being satisfied with the consultation with the nurses, patients are more willing to continue the examination and consultation with the physician, and even some patients can refer to the physician [20]. In some studies, the clinical outcome of patients who were prescribed medication by nurses was similar to medication administered by physicians [31].

Various factors may prevent the implementation of nurse prescribing in some countries, for example, in Iran, including patients, physicians, and officials' distrust of nurses' prescriptions, low awareness of the benefits of nurse prescribing, low self-confidence of nurses, medical staff's critical view on this issue, nurses' fear of responsibility and legal issues, and ignoring the experiences of other countries in this regard [32]. The recent master nursing curriculum alterations in Iran, which indicates the specialization of nursing and the further development of the role to include nurse prescribing, is considered a set in the right direction to enhance the nursing profession. In Iran, master nursing students are required to pass 1–2 units of pharmacology, which can help them in taking on the role of prescribing [1]. Also, in Iran, unlike some countries including the United States, there is no DNP (Doctor of Nursing Practice) degree, and the only doctoral degree is in the form of a Ph.D. During this 4–5-year period, 45 units of study are offered to students, and nursing doctoral students have no pharmacology unit. However, after graduating from nursing schools, as academic staff, they are required to teach theoretical and clinical units that require knowledge of pharmacology [33]. Despite the changes that have occurred in Iran's graduate nursing education curriculum, it seems that these changes are not enough for Iranian nurses to benefit from the prescribing role, and more measures are needed in this regard.

3. Nurse prescribing in Iran

Similar to the UK, in Iran especially in critical care situations, nurses assess the patients and after diagnosing the problem, they wait for the physician to confirm and stamp the diagnosis and prescription taken by the nurse. Therefore, in future possible scenarios for nursing prescription are the works in the UK that have been done. In other words, countries such as Iran (which is in the infancy period) could use the UK experiences to develop their nursing prescription ability. In primary care, which can enable the level of access and cheaper services, or in the clinical areas such as chronic diseases (diabetes, cardiovascular disease, cerebrovascular accidents ...) nurse prescriptions can be started from the list of drugs. And after some time, the independent prescription of drugs will become official from the national formulary, and registered nurses who have at least 3 years of work experience will be allowed to participate in prescription training courses.

Author details

Hamidreza Haririan
Faculty of Nursing and Midwifery, Tabriz University of Medical Sciences, Tabriz, Iran

*Address all correspondence to: houman.haririan@gmail.com

References

[1] Haririan H, Rahmani A, Porter JE, Heidarzadeh M, Azadi A, Faghani S, et al. Nursing students' attitude and preparedness for nurse prescribing and its relationship with self-efficacy. Nurse Education in Practice. 2021;**54**:103126

[2] Gielen SC, Dekker J, Francke AL, Mistiaen P, Kroezen M. The effects of nurse prescribing: A systematic review. International Journal of Nursing Studies. 2014;**51**(7):1048-1061

[3] Klein T, Kaplan L. Prescribing competencies for advanced practice registered nurses. The Journal for Nurse Practitioners. 2010;**6**(2):115-122

[4] Kroezen M, van Dijk L, Groenewegen PP, de Rond M, de Veer AJ, Francke AL. Neutral to positive views on the consequences of nurse prescribing: Results of a national survey among registered nurses, nurse specialists and physicians. International Journal of Nursing Studies. 2014;**51**(4):539-548

[5] Chen-Scarabelli C. Nurse prescribing in the UK. The Lancet. 2002;**360**(9345):1607-1608

[6] Royal College of Nursing. Policy and International Department. RCN Fact Sheet: Nurse prescribing in the UK. RCN; 2012

[7] Cipher DJ, Hooker RS, Guerra P. Prescribing trends by nurse practitioners and physician assistants in the United States. Journal of the American Academy of Nurse practitioners. 2006;**18**(6):291-296

[8] Latter S, Maben J, Myall M, Young A. Evaluating the clinical appropriateness of nurses' prescribing practice: Method development and findings from an expert panel analysis. BMJ Quality and Safety. 2007;**16**(6):415-421

[9] Hobson RJ. Investigation into early implementation of non-medical prescribing in the UK (Doctoral dissertation, University of Bath). 2008

[10] Haririan H. Prescribing: A crucial factor in the professionalization of nursing in Iran. Evidence Based Care. 2016;**5**(4):65-66

[11] Darvishpour A, Joolaee S, Cheraghi MA. Situational analysis of nurse prescribing context in Iran: A qualitative research. Iran Journal of Nursing. 2017;**29**(104):1-6

[12] Shahraki Moghaddam E, Manzari ZS, Ghandehari MZ. The evaluation of nurse, s clinical decision making in intensive care unit at the teaching hospitals of Mashhad. Journal of Sabzevar University of Medical Sciences. 2017;**24**(2):113-107

[13] Nolan P, Bradley E. The role of the nurse prescriber: The views of mental health and non-mental health nurses. Journal of Psychiatric and Mental Health Nursing. 2007;**14**(3):258-266

[14] Darvishpour A. The Analysis of Nurse Prescribing Situation in Iran and Other Countries. Nursing. (Doctoral dissertation). 2014

[15] Babaie L, Haririan H, Rahmani A. Iranian Nurses' attitudes and readiness for nurse prescribing: A cross sectional study. Journal of Holistic Nursing and Midwifery. 2022;**32**(2):116-123

[16] Bowskill D, Timmons S, James V. How do nurse prescribers integrate prescribing in practice: Case studies in primary and secondary

care. Journal of Clinical Nursing. 2013;**22**(13-14):2077-2086

[17] Bradley E, Campbell P, Nolan P. Nurse prescribers: Who are they and how do they perceive their role. Journal of Advanced Nursing. 2005;**51**(5):439-448

[18] Black A, Dawood M. A comparison in independent nurse prescribing and patient group directions by nurse practitioners in the emergency department: A cross sectional review. International Emergency Nursing. 2014;**22**(1):10-17

[19] Lewis-Evans A, Jester R. Nurse prescribers' experiences of prescribing. Journal of Clinical Nursing. 2004;**13**(7):796-805

[20] Gerard K, Tinelli M, Latter S, Smith A, Blenkinsopp A. Patients' valuation of the prescribing nurse in primary care: A discrete choice experiment. Health Expectations. 2015;**18**(6):2223-2235

[21] Luker KA, McHugh GA. Nurse prescribing from the community nurse's perspective. International Journal of Pharmacy Practice. 2002;**10**(4):273-280

[22] Fisher R. Relationships in nurse prescribing in district nursing practice in England: A preliminary investigation. International Journal of Nursing Practice. 2005;**11**(3):102-107

[23] Carey N, Courtenay M, Burke J. Supplementary nurse prescribing for patients with skin conditions: A national questionnaire survey. Journal of Clinical Nursing. 2007;**16**(7):1230-1237

[24] Berry D, Courtenay M, Bersellini E. Attitudes towards, and information needs in relation to, supplementary nurse prescribing in the UK: An empirical study. Journal of Clinical Nursing. 2006;**15**(1):22-28

[25] Afseth JD, Paterson RE. The views of non-medical prescribing students and medical mentors on inter professional competency assessment–a qualitative exploration. Nurse Education Today. 2017;**52**:103-108

[26] Axe S. Numeracy and nurse prescribing: Do the standards achieve their aim? Nurse Education in Practice. 2011;**11**(5):285-287

[27] Lee GA, Fitzgerald L. A clinical internship model for the nurse practitioner program. Nurse Education in Practice. 2008;**8**(6):397-404

[28] Kroezen M, Francke AL, Groenewegen PP, van Dijk L. Nurse prescribing of medicines in Western European and Anglo-Saxon countries: A survey on forces, conditions and jurisdictional control. International Journal of Nursing Studies. 2012;**49**(8):1002-1012

[29] Courtenay M, Carey N. Nurse independent prescribing and nurse supplementary prescribing practice: National survey. Journal of Advanced Nursing. 2008;**61**(3):291-299

[30] Carberry M, Connelly S, Murphy J. A prospective audit of a nurse independent prescribing within critical care. Nursing in Critical Care. 2013;**18**(3):135-141

[31] Stuart J. How can Nurses Address Generalist/Specialist/Nursing Requirements of the Urban/Rural Population of Southland. 2003

[32] Sajjadi M, Khoshnazar T, Shareinia H, Rassouli M. A review on

prescribing in nursing. Iranian Journal of Nursing Research. 2016;**10**(4):67-75

[33] Borzou SR, Oshvandi K, Cheraghi F, Moayed MS. Comparative study of nursing PhD education system and curriculum in Iran and John Hopkins school of nursing. Education Strategies in Medical Sciences. 2016;**9**(3):194-205

Chapter 11

Perspective Chapter: Adaptation of the Quality-Caring Model to Hospitalized School-Aged Children and Their Parents

Fernanda Loureiro, Vanessa Antunes and Zaida Charepe

Abstract

The development of nursing theory improves nursing practice and consequently the health of those who receive nursing care. This chapter aims to describe the process of adaptation of the quality-caring model to hospitalized school-aged children and their parents. A mixed methods study in four phases was outlined. The study integrated a literature review (phase 1); the application of surveys to hospitalized children and their parents (phase 2); a Delphi panel with nurses as experts (phase 3); and the adaptation of the quality-caring model (phase 4). Participants included hospitalized children (n = 252), their parents (n = 251), and nurses (round 1 n = 47; round 2 n = 42). National Data Protection Commission provided authorization for the study as well as the ethics committee from six health institutions where the study was applied. Findings allowed the identification of key aspects valued by children, parents, and nurses, such as information, family involvement, play, distraction, and communication. The adapted model integrates fundamental aspects of children's hospitalization and is focused on satisfaction with care as an outcome of nursing care.

Keywords: child, hospitalization, patient satisfaction, pediatric nursing, family centred care

1. Introduction

Family centered care has been considered the best practice in pediatric hospitalized care [1]. This approach to child health care lies in the belief that the emotional and developmental needs of children are best achieved when families are integrated and involved in care [2, 3]. Despite, it has been used as a philosophy of care world-wide [4] there is still a lack of research that proves its greater effectiveness in comparison to other perspectives [5]. Further theoretical conceptions are applied to hospitalized children and have been reported in the literature such as the theory of basic human needs [6–8], the theory of human care [9], or the comfort theory [10]. The quality-caring model [11] is also identified as particularly suitable since it is based on Watson's [12], King's [13], and Donabedian's [14] work. This model highlights the importance of the nursing profession and has successively been implemented in pediatric hospital settings [15].

The seeds of this model were sown throughout considerations regarding nursing interventions and while exploring outcomes variables of patient satisfaction [16]. The purpose of this model is to guide professional practice and to provide a foundation for nursing research. The model was initially developed in 2003 [17] and later updated in 2020 with four main concepts that include humans in relationship; relationship-centered professional encounters; feeling "cared for"; and self-advancing systems [16]. The revised version accentuates the link between caring relationships and quality of care where patient satisfaction is integrated. A major proposition of this model is that relationships are important to care and positively contribute to outcomes in clients, families, care providers, and ultimately the health system.

Theories are embraced by nurses to guide and create a practice that is meaningful to them. Also, the development and study of nursing theory improve nursing practice and consequently the health and quality of life of those who receive nursing care [18]. The main aim of this chapter is to describe the process of adaptation of the revised quality-caring model [16] to hospitalized school-aged children and their parents based on research findings.

2. Methods

This is a mixed-method study that occurred in four phases. The focus was on nursing care provided to hospitalized school-aged children and their parents. The study was applied in hospitals and all perspectives were considered, namely, from children, parents, and nurses. National Data Protection Commission provided authorization for the study (1644/2015) as well as ethics committees in each of the institutions where the study was undertaken. A brief description of each phase is presented for contextualization purposes. In this chapter, we are addressing the results from phase 4.

2.1 Phase 1: literature review

Initially, an extensive literature review was performed that included the clarification of patient satisfaction with the nursing care concept [19]; an integrative literature review [20] to identify children's satisfaction with nursing care during hospitalization [21]; and a scoping review [22] to identify nursing theoretical conceptions used in hospitalized child care [5] that led us to the selection of the quality-caring model [17] in its revised version [16].

2.2 Phase 2: evaluating satisfaction with care: children's and parent perspectives

In phase 2, the aim was to identify children's and parents' satisfaction with nursing care. An observational, cross-sectional, and exploratory-descriptive study was performed with a non-probabilistic and accidental sample of 252 children aged 7–11 years and 251 parents from 6 health institutions.

Regarding children, data were collected through the Child Care Quality at Hospital (CCQH) [23] survey. The instrument has 49 items allocated within three domains: nurses' characteristics, nurses' activities, and the nursing environment. The last two items are open-ended sentences where children are asked to complete the following phrases: "in my opinion the best thing about the hospital is ..." and "in my opinion the worst thing about the hospital is ...". Original instrument development occurred in three phases: phase I version developed based on the literature review and submitted to an expert panel; phase II instrument application to 41 children and appraised by 19 nurses; and phase III instrument's psychometric characteristics were assessed (factor analysis and internal consistency through Cronbach's alpha: nurses' characteristics (0.557), nurses' activities (0.809), and nursing environment (0.761)) [23]. For this study, the instrument was translated and validated into Portuguese [24].

Parents' perspective was evaluated with the application of the Citizen Satisfaction with Nursing Care (CSNC) survey after validation to this particular population [25]. This survey assesses citizens' satisfaction with nursing care experiences and includes sociodemographic data, the Nursing Care Experiences scale with 28 items (seven-item Likert scale), the Opinions on Nursing Care scale, with 19 items (five-item Likert scale), and two open questions: "What aspects of nursing care could be improved?" and "Do you have any other comments?"

Both data were submitted to statistical analysis through SPSS statistical tool (version 24.0).

2.3 Phase 3: nurse's perspectives

In phase 3, the purpose was to identify strategies described by nurses that aimed at increasing children's and parents' satisfaction with nursing care. Data were collected through a Delphi panel and a total of 90 nurses working in the institutions where phase 2 was applied, with at least 3 years of experience, were contacted. Data analysis included content analysis [26] in round 1 and statistical analysis in round 2 considering criteria for determining the degree of consensus previously established.

2.4 Phase 4: proposal for nursing care

In the final phase results from previous phases were incorporated into a proposal for nursing practice. This proposal included a synthesis of nursing interventions and nursing activities that promote satisfaction as well as a proposal to adapt the revised quality-caring model [16] to this particular setting and population. This process will be further explained in the next sections.

3. Results

As previously mentioned, the main results from each phase will be presented for contextualization purposes.

3.1 Phase 1: literature review

The conceptual analysis of patient satisfaction with the nursing care concept comprised Walker and Avant's method [27] as well as an integrative literature review that included a sample of 19 studies. This allowed the identification of concept antecedents and consequences concerning patients and nurses. The definition of empirical references to the essential concept attributes allowed an operational definition of patient satisfaction with nursing care in the hospital. It was defined as a personal opinion that confronts perceived needs, expectations of care, and experiences of care received in professional, personal, and environmental domains [19].

The integrative literature review that aimed at synthesizing current knowledge about school-aged children's satisfaction with nursing care in hospital settings [21] was performed with the steps suggested by Whittemore and Knafl [20]. The sample of 23 studies showed that children's perspective is yet poorly understood. From the article's analysis, three themes were identified: expectations of nursing care, experiences with nursing care, and strategies to improve satisfaction during hospitalization.

Additionally, a scoping review complemented this phase. Tricco et al. [22] suggested steps were followed to identify nursing theoretical conceptions used in the particular setting of hospitalized children [5]. From the 21 articles selected, it was possible to identify a range of theoretical conceptions. They were adapted from already existing conceptions, such as the synergy model [28], or specifically developed for this population and setting such as the child transitional communication model [29]. From the total of ten conceptions identified, the quality-caring model [17] was chosen, in its revised version [16], due to its appropriateness to the setting, populations, and concept of this study.

3.2 Phase 2: evaluating satisfaction with care: children and parent perspectives

Results from the application of the CCQH [23], in its Portuguese version [24], showed that children were generally satisfied.

Psychometric properties were measured to determine the instrument's reliability and validity. Exploratory factor analysis of main components with Varimax rotation was used for construct validity as well as Cronbach's alpha coefficient for internal consistency (values between 0.66 and 0.82). Psychometric characteristics assured the Portuguese version's reliability and validity [24].

The sample (n = 252) included mainly boys (52.8%, n = 133) with average age of 8.9 years (SD = 1.4), most children had surgical or medical unscheduled admissions (84,6%; n = 209) and 15,4% (n = 38) had scheduled hospital admission. Global nursing care (1–5) was rated with a score of 4.51 (SD = 0.645). Sociodemographic factors did not have an effect on overall satisfaction in our sample. Most valued aspects included nurses being "nice" (nurses' characteristics), "listening" (nurses' activities), and the nursing environment. Open-ended questions were submitted to content analysis [26]. Children recognized "people" (f = 113), "physical environment" (f = 81), "activities" (f = 49), "outcomes" (f = 32), and "food" (f = 10) from 209 answers as best experiences. "Feelings" (f = 59), "activities" (f = 54), "food" (f = 48), "environment" (f = 15), and "outcomes" (f = 12) were identified as worst experiences from 203 answers [30].

Regarding parents, the application of the CSNC survey also revealed satisfaction with nursing care. Psychometric properties of reliability (Cronbach's alpha coefficient) and content validity (exploratory factor analysis with principal components and orthogonal Varimax rotation) were assessed. Adequate psychometric characteristics were found (Cronbach's alpha of 0.92) ensuring instrument reliability and validity [25].

The sample (n = 251) includes mainly women (83.7%, n = 210) with average age of 37.65 years (SD = 6.3). On the scale of "nursing care experiences", parents felt "at ease with nurses" (76.7%, n = 193), "saw nurses as friends" (53%, n = 133) and thought that "nurses promoted a pleasant atmosphere" (77.6%, n = 195), so most parents would return to the unit if the child needed it (76.9%, n = 193). On the scale of "nursing care opinion", parents considered that "a nurse was always around when needed" (73.3%, n = 184), frequently questioning if the child was well (74.9%, n = 188) and reassuring family and friends (66.2%, n = 174) [31]. When asked "which aspects of nursing care could be improved?" most parents did not respond to this question (53.4%, n = 134). Among the total respondents (n = 117), five categories were identified: "satisfaction" (f = 71), "personal domain" (f = 22), "environmental domain" (f = 18) "professional domain" (f = 1), and "nursing assignment" (f = 6) [32].

3.3 Phase 3: nurse's perspectives

In this phase, nurse's perspective was sought. Delphi technique [33] was applied in two rounds and allowed the identification of nursing interventions to promote an increase in children's and parents' satisfaction [34]. The invitation to participate in the study was sent to a total of 90 nurses in each round.

3.3.1 Round 1

Of the 90 nurses that were initially contacted 47 nurses (response rate 52%) participated in round 1. Open-ended questions were placed that addressed strategies to promote satisfaction in children and parents and the difficulties/constraints to implement these strategies. Participant's ages ranged between 25 and 60 years (average age of 38.5 years; SD = 7.7) and 3–38 years of professional experience in child health. From content analysis [26] to answers from round 1, a total of 25 nursing interventions were identified. Nursing Intervention Classification taxonomy [35] was integrated into this analysis. In round 2, results from round 1 were presented to comprehend which strategies were considered significant by nurses.

3.3.2 Round 2

In this round, the same 90 nurses were contacted. 42 nurses (response rate 47%) participated in round 2 and all interventions reached consensus. Participant's ages ranged between 26 and 61 years (average age 40.1; SD = 8.5) and a professional experience between 6 and 38 years with an average of 16 years (SD = 8.2). Regarding interventions directed to children, 13 interventions were considered in the following areas: information transmission; family involvement; play strategies; children's distraction; maintenance of children's routine; care environment control; humor; and articulation with community resources and children's admission [34]. Regarding parents, 12 interventions reach consensus in round 2 in different areas, namely, family involvement; information transmission; family support; communication; children's admission; and family union strategies [34].

Difficulties/constraints to implement these interventions included for both children, and parents: lack of resources (time, human, and materials); institutional and organizational aspects; communicational approach; and previous hospitalization experiences.

3.4 Phase 4: proposal for nursing care

The final phase of this study incorporated results from previous phases into a proposal for nursing practice considering the satisfaction of hospitalized school-aged children and their parents. This proposal integrates a synthesis of interventions, a set of orientations to nursing practice, and the adaptation of the revised quality-caring model [16] as a result of all study phases. The set of orientations was proposed as general topics to address that include: a systematic evaluation of school-aged children and their parent's satisfaction with nursing care with valid surveys at every 3 months; inclusion of family members that are relevant to children in satisfaction evaluation; inclusion of a space for additional comments in satisfaction surveys; results of these evaluations should be disclosed for all health care teams; implementation of individualized care sensitive to each child and family; entertainment should be effectively incorporated in nursing care; improvement of communication with children and parents; use of satisfaction survey results to improve nursing care; and institutional policies that aim at the improvement of hospital experience and implementation of nursing interventions and activities that promote children and parent satisfaction.

Finally, the adaptation of the revised quality-caring model [16] that included results from all phases is further explained in the discussion section.

4. Discussion

Nursing theory development is a nursing research priority [36]. Particularly, theory-guided practice is considered by Saleh [37] as the future of nursing as a way to provide effective, efficient, and holistic care. To do so, nurses must rely on theoretical principles to apply the plan of care [37]. In this chapter, we present an adaptation of a nursing model based on research results.

The first main component of the revised quality-caring model [16] is humans in a relationship which refers to the notion that humans are multidimensional beings. This component considers human characteristics and their influence on nursing interventions. In this study, personal characteristics of nurse were considered since they are identified as important both in the literature review [21] and in the results from phase 2 [31]. Children value personal characteristics such as being friendly and approachable [38] or being treated with respect [39]. Parents mentioned these characteristics as something desirable that can be enhanced to improve satisfaction [32]. Interestingly, nurses did not identify any intervention that was focused on this area of improvement.

Previous experiences of hospitalization were mentioned by parents, children, and nurses as an important factor that can affect satisfaction with care. Also, in literature, previous experiences appear relevant [40] as well as socio-demographic factors [41]. Demographic factors appeared as particularly relevant given the different development characteristics of children regarding age and gender. Age is identified as an important factor [42]; however, in our study, there was no link between children's age and satisfaction.

In this population and setting, pediatric internment units also resources such as toys, environment of care, and resource adequacy must be considered given the characteristics of school-aged children. The importance of play and toys in pediatric care is well documented in the literature [43, 44] and was expected to appear as an important factor in all phases of this study. Similarly, the environment of care in physical, emotional, and social dimensions was also found in literature and in results from phases 2 and 3 of this study. The adequacy of resources was primarily mentioned by parents [32] and nurses [34]. Parents highlight the importance of having enough nurses and time when implementing care plans and nurses highlighted how time could be a constraint to implement interventions that improve satisfaction.

The second component of the revised quality caring model [16] is named relationship-centered professional encounters. In this component, admission care

DOI: http://dx.doi.org/10.5772/intechopen.110743

appeared as a relevant moment. In our study, both parents and nurses mentioned the importance of having a satisfying experience when first entering the hospital unit. Also, respect appears repeatedly as the factor that most influences satisfaction [45] and was identified by parents in our study. Other aspects added were communication and information, family involvement, play/distraction/humor, union and family support, and pain management. All these aspects were identified by children, parents, and nurses as central to a satisfying hospitalization and central to relationships with nurses. Time management is a particular area that appears in the literature and was highlighted by all participants. Nurses identified time management as a constraint; however, no strategies concerning this theme were suggested.

Play and humor were also identified by all participants as aspects that are central to children's hospitalizations and influence satisfaction with care. A good sense of humor is considered a desirable nurse characteristic by hospitalized children [42] since it can positively reduce tension and facilitate approachability, comfort, and dialog [46]. The importance of play to children's well-being is unquestionable but also to family and health teams [47].

The third component feeling "cared for" is identified as a positive emotion and an important antecedent to quality health outcomes [16] where satisfaction is included. Pain management, satisfaction with care, and knowledge/information were identified as relevant factors. Pain is also a central theme in children's hospitalizations that was mentioned by all participants. It is identified as one of the worst experiences for children [30] and good pain management is an expectation for both children [48] and parents [49].

The last component of the revised quality caring model is self-advancing systems and is identified as something that appears gradually as a reflection of "dynamic positive progress that enhances the systems' well-being" [16]. Implications in the health care system include an intention to re-use services and resource adequacy. The link between satisfaction with care and these two factors has already been established in the literature [50]. When patients' perspective is sought and taken into consideration, nursing care is more centered on patient real needs and therefore more satisfying [51]. Articulation with community resources was also mentioned by both parents and nurses.

5. Conclusion

The adapted model integrates fundamental aspects of children's hospitalization and is focused on satisfaction with care as an outcome of nursing care. It maintains the belief that persons, in this case, children and parents, are multi-contextual beings that are linked to a larger and diversified world. This adaptation allowed the identification of aspects of nursing care that are relevant to this population and setting. By doing so the adapted model integrates evidence from research that does benefit children and parents.

Acknowledgements

The authors would like to thank the nurses, parents, and all the children who accepted to participate in the study as well as the institutions that authorized this study.

Conflict of interest

The authors declare no conflict of interest.

Appendices and nomenclature

CCQH	Children Care Quality at Hospital
CSNC	Citizen Satisfaction with Nursing Care

Author details

Fernanda Loureiro[1*], Vanessa Antunes[1] and Zaida Charepe[2]

1 Egas Moniz School of Health and Science, Multidisciplinary Research Center of Egas Moniz (CiiEM), Caparica, Portugal

2 Portuguese Catholic University, Centre for Interdisciplinary Research in Health (CIIS), Lisbon, Portugal

*Address all correspondence to: floureiro@egasmoniz.edu.pt

References

[1] Coyne I, Holmström I, Söderbäck M. Centeredness in healthcare: A concept synthesis of family-centered care, person-centered care and child-centered care. Journal of Pediatric Nursing. 2018;**42**:45-56. DOI: 10.1016/j.pedn.2018.07.001

[2] Watts R, Zhou H, Shields L, Taylor M, Munns A, Ngune I. Family-centered care for hospitalized children aged 0-12 years: A systematic review of qualitative studies. JBI Database Syst Rev Implement Reports. 2014;**12**:204-283. DOI: 10.11124/jbisrir-2014-1683

[3] Shields L, Zhou H, Taylor M, Hunter J, Munns A, Watts R. Family-centred care for hospitalised children aged 0-12 years: A systematic review of quasi-experimental studies. JBI Library System Review. 2012;**10**:2559-2592. DOI: 10.11124/jbisrir-2012-32

[4] Kuo DZ, Houtrow AJ, Arango P, Kuhlthau KA, Simmons JM, Neff JM. Family-centered care: Current applications and future directions in pediatric health care. Maternal and Child Health Journal. 2012;**16**:297-305. DOI: 10.1007/s10995-011-0751-7

[5] Loureiro FM, dos Antunes AV, Charepe ZB. Theoretical nursing conceptions in hospitalized child care: Scoping review. Revista Brasileira de Enfermagem. 2021;**74**:1-11. DOI: 10.1590/0034-7167-2020-0265

[6] Dantas AMN, de Silva K, Nóbrega MML. Validation of nursing diagnoses, interventions and outcomes in a pediatric clinic. Revista Brasileira de Enfermagem. 2018;**71**:80-88. DOI: 10.1590/0034-7167-2016-0647

[7] Marques DKA, de Silva K, Nóbrega MML. Escolares hospitalizados: proposta de um instrumento para coleta de dados à luz da teoria de Horta. Rev Gaúcha Enferm. 2016;**2016**:37. DOI: 10.1590/1983-1447.2016.esp.2016-0038

[8] Santos P, Silva L, Depianti J, Cursino E, Ribeiro C. Nursing care through the perception of hospitalized children. Revista Brasileira de Enfermagem. 2016;**69**:646-653. DOI: 10.1590/0034-7167.2016690405i

[9] dos Santos MR, Bousso RS, Vendramim P, Baliza MF, Misko MD, Silva L. The practice of nurses caring for families of pediatric inpatients in light of Jean Watson. Rev da Esc Enferm da USP. 2014;**48**:80-86. DOI: 10.1590/S0080-623420140000600012

[10] Kolcaba K, DiMarco MA. Comfort theory and its application to pediatric nursing. Pediatric Nursing 2015;31:187-194. Available from: http://www.ncbi.nlm.nih.gov/pubmed/16060582 [Accessed: 4 July 2019]

[11] Duffy JR. Joanne Duffy's quality-caring model©. In: Smith M, Parker M, editors. Nursing Teories and Nursing Practice. Philadelphia: F.A. Davis Company; 2015. pp. 393-429

[12] Watson J. Nursing: The Philosophy and Science of Caring. Boulder: University Press of Colorado; 2008

[13] King IM. King's theory of goal attainment in practice. Nursing Science Quarterly. 1997;**10**:180-185. DOI: 10.1177/089431849701000411

[14] Donabedian A. An Introduction to Quality Assurance in Health Care. New York: Oxford University Press; 2003

[15] Edmundson E. The quality caring nursing model: A journey to selection

and implementation. Journal of Pediatric Nursing. 2012;**27**:411-415. DOI: 10.1016/j.pedn.2011.09.007

[16] Duffy JR. Joanne Duffy's quality-caring model. In: Smith M, editor. Nursing Theories and Nursing Practice. 5th ed. Philadelphia: F.A. Davis Company; 2020. pp. 383-398

[17] Duffy JR, Hoskins LM. The quality-caring model©. Advances in Nursing Science. 2003;**26**:77-88. DOI: 10.1097/00012272-200301000-00010

[18] Smith M, Parker M. Nursing theory and the discipline of nursing. In: Smith MC, Gullett DL, editors. Nursing Theories and Nursing Practice. 5th ed. Philadelphia: F. A. Davis; 2020. pp. 3-16

[19] Loureiro FM, Charepe ZB. Satisfação do Paciente com os Cuidados de Enfermagem no Hospital: Análise do Conceito. Cad Saúde. 2018;**10**:23-29. DOI: 10.34632/cadernosdesaude.2018.6787

[20] Whittemore R, Knafl K. The integrative review: Updated methodology. Journal of Advanced Nursing. 2005;**52**:546-553

[21] Loureiro F, Figueiredo MH, Charepe Z. Nursing care satisfaction from school-aged children's perspective: An integrative review. International Journal of Nursing Practice. 2019;**2019**:25. DOI: 10.1111/ijn.12764

[22] Tricco AC, Lillie E, Zarin W, O'Brien KK, Colquhoun H, Levac D, et al. PRISMA extension for scoping reviews (PRISMA-ScR): Checklist and explanation. Annals of Internal Medicine. 2018;**169**:467. DOI: 10.7326/M18-0850

[23] Pelander T, Leino-Kilpi H, Katajisto J. The quality of paediatric nursing care: Developing the child care quality at hospital instrument for children. Journal of Advanced Nursing. 2009;**65**:443-453. DOI: 10.1111/j.1365-2648.2008.04875.x

[24] Loureiro FM, Araújo BR, Charepe ZB. Adaptation and validation of the instrument ' children care quality at hospital ' for Portuguese. Aquichan. 2019;**19**:1-13

[25] Loureiro F, Araújo B, Charepe Z. Validação da Escala de Satisfação do Cidadão com Cuidados de Enfermagem para pais de crianças hospitalizadas. Rev Enferm Ref. 2021;**5**:1-8. DOI: 10.12707/RV20062

[26] Bardin L. Content Analysis. Lisboa: Edições; 2013. p. 70

[27] Walker LO, Avant KC. Strategies for Theory Construction in Nursing. 5th Editio. London: Pearson; 2014. Available from: http://www.amazon.com/Strategies-Theory-Construction-Nursing-Edition/dp/0132156881 [Accessed: 3 Sep 2014]

[28] Curley MA. Patient-nurse synergy: Optimizing patients' outcomes. American Journal of Critical Care 1998;7:64-72. Available from: http://www.ncbi.nlm.nih.gov/pubmed/9429685 [Accessed 4 Mar 2020]

[29] Lambert V, Glacken M, McCarron M. Communication between children and health professionals in a child hospital setting: A child transitional communication model. Journal of Advanced Nursing. 2011;**67**:569-582. DOI: 10.1111/j.1365-2648.2010.05511.x

[30] Loureiro FM, dos Antunes AV, Pelander T, Charepe ZB. The experience of school-aged children with hospitalisation. Journal of Clinical Nursing. 2020;**2020**:15574. DOI: 10.1111/jocn.15574

[31] Loureiro F, Charepe Z. Hospitalization of school age children - Parents satisfaction with nursing care. Translational Research and Innovation in Human and Health Science. 2018;**2018**:260

[32] Loureiro F, Charepe Z. How to improve nursing care? Perspectives of hospitalized school aged children parents. Annals of Medicine. 2018;**2018**:S160. DOI: 10.1080/07853890.2018.1427445

[33] Keeney S, Hasson F, Mckenna H. The Delphi Technique in Nursing and Health Research. 1a. ed. Oxford: Wiley-Blackwell; 2011

[34] Loureiro FM, Charepe ZB. Strategies for increase satisfaction with nursing care in hospitalized children: A Delphi study. Enferm Glob. 2021;**20**:161-175

[35] Butcher HK, editor. Nursing Interventions Classification. 7th ed. Missouri: Elsevier; 2018

[36] Hopia H, Heikkilä J. Nursing research priorities based on CINAHL database: A scoping review. Nursing Open. 2020;7:483-494. DOI: 10.1002/nop2.428

[37] Saleh US. Theory guided practice in nursing. Journal of Nursig Research Practise. 2018;2:18. Available from: https://www.pulsus.com/scholarly-articles/theory-guided-practice-in-nursing.pdf

[38] Fletcher T, Glasper A, Prudhoe G, Battrick C, Coles L, Weaver K, et al. Building the future: Children's views on nurses and hospital care. The British Journal of Nursing. 2011;**20**:39-45. DOI: 10.12968/bjon.2011.20.1.39

[39] Pelander T, Leino-Kilpi H. Quality in pediatric nursing care: Children's expectations. Issues in Comprehensive Pediatric Nursing. 2004;**27**:139-151. DOI: 10.1080/01460860490497778

[40] Pelander T, Leino-Kilpi H, Katajisto J. Quality of Pediatric nursing Care in Finland. Journal of Nursing Care Quality. 2007;**22**:185-194. DOI: 10.1097/01.NCQ.0000263110.38591.9a

[41] Quintana JM, González N, Bilbao A, Aizpuru F, Escobar A, Esteban C, et al. Predictors of patient satisfaction with hospital health care. BMC Health Services Research. 2006;**6**:102. DOI: 10.1186/1472-6963-6-102

[42] Comparcini D, Simonetti V, Tomietto M, Leino-Kilpi H, Pelander T, Cicolini G. Children's perceptions about the quality of Pediatric nursing care: A large Multicenter cross-sectional study. Journal of Nursing Scholarship. 2018;**50**:287-295. DOI: 10.1111/jnu.12381

[43] Marcinowicz L, Abramowicz P, Zarzycka D, Abramowicz M, Konstantynowicz J. How hospitalized children and parents perceive nurses and hospital amenities: A qualitative descriptive study in Poland. Journal of Child Health Care. 2016;**20**:120-128. DOI: 10.1177/1367493514551313

[44] Boztepe H, Çınar S, Ay A. School-age children's perception of the hospital experience. Journal of Child Health Care. 2017;**21**:162-170. DOI: 10.1177/1367493517690454

[45] Otani K, Herrmann P, a, Kurz RS. Improving patient satisfaction in hospital care settings. Health Services Management Research. 2011;**24**:163-169. DOI: 10.1258/hsmr.2011.011008

[46] Petronio-Coia BJ, Schwartz-Barcott D. A description of approachable nurses: An exploratory study, the voice of the hospitalized child. Journal of

Pediatric Nursing. 2020;**54**:18-23. DOI: 10.1016/j.pedn.2020.05.011

[47] Gama DON, Silva DO, Pereira RB, Camarão YPHC. A importância do lúdico no contexto da hospitalização infantil. Rev Enferm UFPE line. 2018;**12**:3484. DOI: 10.5205/1981-8963-v12i12a234923p3484-3491-2018

[48] Schalkers I, Dedding CWM, Bunders JFG. "[I would like] a place to be alone, other than the toilet" - Children's perspectives on paediatric hospital care in the Netherlands. Health Expectations. 2015;**18**:2066-2078

[49] Matziou V, Boutopoulou B, Chrysostomou A, Vlachioti E, Mantziou T, Petsios K. Parents' satisfaction concerning their child's hospital care. Japan Journal of Nursing Science. 2011;**8**:163-173. DOI: 10.1111/j.1742-7924.2010.00171.x

[50] You L, Aiken LH, Sloane DM, Liu K, He G, Hu Y, et al. Hospital nursing, care quality, and patient satisfaction: Cross-sectional surveys of nurses and patients in hospitals in China and Europe. International Journal of Nursing Studies. 2013;**50**:154-161. DOI: 10.1016/j.ijnurstu.2012.05.003

[51] Ng JHY, Luk BHK. Patient satisfaction: Concept analysis in the healthcare context. Patient Education and Counseling. 2019;**102**:790-796. DOI: 10.1016/j.pec.2018.11.013